Praise for *Secrets of the World's Healthiest Children*

'This is a great set of principles that are solidly based
and yet simple'

Dr Walter Willett, Chair, Department of Nutrition,
Harvard School of Public Health, one of the world's
leading nutritionists, on this book's key tips

'A meticulously researched book full of valuable practical
advice, *Secrets of the World's Healthiest Children* deserves a
place on every parent's bookshelf'

Dr Lucy Cooke, Honorary Senior Research Associate,
Department of Epidemiology and Public Health,
University College London

Secrets of the World's Healthiest Children

Naomi Moriyama
and
William Doyle

piatkus

PIATKUS

First published in Great Britain in 2015 by Piatkus

1 3 5 7 9 10 8 6 4 2

Copyright © Naomi Moriyama and William Doyle 2015

The moral right of the authors has been asserted.

A CIP catalogue record for this book
is available from the British Library.

ISBN 978-0-349-40748-7

Typeset in Calluna and The Sans by M Rules
Printed and bound in Great Britain by
Clays Ltd, St Ives plc

Papers used by Piatkus are from well-managed forests
and other responsible sources.

MIX
Paper from
responsible sources
FSC® C104740

Piatkus
An imprint of
Little, Brown Book Group
Carmelite House
50 Victoria Embankment
London EC4Y 0DZ

An Hachette UK Company
www.hachette.co.uk

www.piatkus.co.uk

To our parents, Chizuko, Shigeo,
Marilou and William and our son Brendan

About the authors

Naomi Moriyama is the co-author of *The Times* bestseller *Japanese Women Don't Get Old or Fat*, which was hailed by the *Washington Post* as 'a delicious way to stay healthy' and by the American Dietetic Association as 'a dietary plan that is based on sound science and offers straightforward dietary advice that works'. The book was translated into 19 languages, triggered the sequel *The Japan Diet* and was a *Wall Street Journal International* Best New Year Diet Book.

Naomi has served as chief marketing consultant for Ralph Lauren Japan, as director of marketing at HBO in New York, and as account executive at Grey Advertising in Tokyo and New York, working on the Procter & Gamble and Kraft General Foods accounts. Her first job was as a translator at Tokyo Disneyland. She grew up in Tokyo and on her grandparents' farm in rural Japan. She has been a judge on The Food Network's acclaimed *Iron Chef America* programme, and a guest on the US leading network TV programmes *The Today Show*, *The View* and *Dr Oz*.

Naomi lives in New York City with her seven-year-old son and her husband and co-author, William Doyle.

William Doyle is an award-winning, *New York Times* bestselling author, and co-author with Naomi Moriyama of *Japanese Women Don't Get Old or Fat* and *The Japan Diet*. He has authored or co-authored 14 books, served as director of original programming for HBO, and been producer for the HBO, A&E and PBS TV networks. He has been selected a Fulbright Scholar for 2015–16.

Contents

PART 3 Japanese Inspirations for Family Meals

An Important Note to the Reader

This publication is intended to provide helpful and informative material on the subjects addressed. It is sold with the understanding that the authors and publisher are not engaged in rendering medical, health or any other kind of personal or professional services in the book. The reader should consult his or her own health-care professional before adopting any of the suggestions in this book or drawing inferences from it.

This book includes the opinions of a cross-section of experts, but every child is different, every family is different, and issues about your children's health should always be addressed in consultation with a fully qualified medical professional such as a medical doctor, registered dietician and/or psychiatrist.

This book is not intended in any way to be a substitute for professional medical advice, diagnosis or treatment. Never disregard professional medical advice or delay in seeking it because of something you have read in this book. The author and publisher specifically disclaim all responsibility for any liability, injury, loss or risk, personal or otherwise, which is incurred as a consequence, directly or indirectly, of the use and application of any of the contents of this book.

Acknowledgements

We thank Claudia Connal and Jillian Stewart at Little, Brown; our literary agent, Mel Berger of WME; our copy editor, Jan Cutler; and our families in the United States and Japan.

We also thank the medical, scientific and academic experts who reviewed and commented on our key recommendations, including: Dr Walter Willett, MD, Chair, Department of Nutrition, Harvard School of Public Health; Dr Lucy Cooke, PhD, Honorary Senior Research Associate, University College London and Great Ormond Street Hospital; Prof. Louise Baur, MD, Professor of Paediatrics and Child Health, University of Sydney Associate Dean, The Children's Hospital at Westmead Clinical School, University of Sydney, Professor, Sydney School of Public Health, University of Sydney, Consultant Paediatrician, Weight Management Services, The Children's Hospital at Westmead; Dr David L. Katz, MD, MPH, FACPM, FACP, Director, Yale University Prevention Research Center, Griffin Hospital Clinical Instructor in Medicine Yale University School of Medicine, President, American College of Lifestyle Medicine, Editor-in-Chief, Childhood Obesity; Dr Boyd Swinburn MBChB, MD, FRACP, Professor of Population Nutrition and Global Health, University of Auckland, Alfred Deakin Professor, Co-Director, WHO Collaborating Centre for Obesity Prevention, Deakin University, Melbourne; Professor Leann L. Birch, PhD; William P. 'Bill' Flatt, Professor, Department of Foods and Nutrition, The University of Georgia; Dr Yoni Freedhoff, MD, assistant professor of family medicine at the University of Ottawa, founder and medical director of the Bariatric Medical Institute dedicated to non-surgical weight management; Dr Rosemary Stanton, OAM, BSc, C Nutr/Diet, G Dip Admin, PhD (Hon), APD; Professor

Anoop Misra, Chairman, Fortis-C-DOC Centre of Excellence for Diabetes, Metabolic Diseases and Endocrinology, Chairman, National Diabetes, Obesity and Cholesterol Foundation, Director, Diabetes and Metabolic Diseases, Diabetes Foundation (India), New Delhi; Dr Seema Gulati, Head, Nutrition Research Group, Centre of Nutrition & Metabolic Research (C-NET), National Diabetes, Obesity and Cholesterol Foundation (N-DOC), Chief Project Officer, Diabetes Foundation (India).

We also thank Charlotte Pinter; Robert Waterhouse; Dr Craig Yancho; Dr Kenneth Pecota; and Ms Ellen Leventry, Cornell University, College of Agriculture and Life Sciences; and the many Japanese mothers we interviewed for this book, including Mitsuko Oka, Chisato Hasegawa, Erika Hashimoto, Misato Hayashi, Jyunko Ishikawa, Takako Komatsu, Miho Sonoshita, Maki Yoneta and Namiko Yoshino.

A father's favour overtops the mountain; a mother's kindness is deeper than the sea.

When you have children, then you will comprehend your parents' kindness.

The parents can see best the character of the child.

To pamper children is to desert them.

If you would bend the tree, do it while it's young.

The spirit of a three-year-old will last until a hundred.

He who has his stomach full only 80 per cent will not need a doctor.

It is the way of the world that things do not turn out as expected.

Life is like a dream of spring.

Japanese sayings

Introduction
Japanese Children are Winning the World Health Olympics

A far, far distant land is paradise I've heard them say;
but those who want to go can reach there in a day.

Japanese poem

Something beautiful is happening on a chain of rocky islands in the Pacific Ocean. Tens of millions of children are winning the World Health Olympics. And they have some life-changing lessons for the rest of the world.

In December 2012, an international team of researchers backed by the Bill and Melinda Gates Foundation published the results of a major worldwide health study in the prestigious medical journal the *Lancet*. Titled the 'Global Burden of Disease Study', you could also call it the 'World Health Olympics', as it is the most detailed nation-by-nation analysis of health and healthy life expectancy ever attempted.

The researchers ranked the world's 187 nations by projected healthy life expectancy, or HALE, which synthesises all the forces of health, mortality, disease, risk factors and other health indicators, as they appear today, into a single 'snapshot' ranking as of one point in time. According to Haidong Wang, assistant professor at the University of Washington School Department of Global Health, and a researcher for the Global Burden of Disease

Study, 'HALE is the average number of years that a child born in a particular nation today can expect to live in "full health" assuming she or he will experience the currently observed age specific mortality and morbidity throughout her or his lifetime, which excludes the years lived in less-than-full health due to disease, hospitalisation, and/or injury.'

In the midst of a global obesity epidemic that is engulfing multitudes of children around the planet, damaging their health, shortening their lives and unleashing a wave of future suffering on them, the *Lancet* study uncovered a shining beacon of hope. The study revealed the nation with the number-one healthiest life expectancy for both men and women. That nation is Japan. It beats its closest competitor by a full two years.

According to the study, if you are a child born in Japan today, you are projected to have a longer healthy life than a child born in any other country on earth – you are projected to enjoy both the longest life and the healthiest life.

How did the UK do? It was not even in the top 20. It came in at number 23, just ahead of Chile and Portugal. Here are the results of the 'World Healthy Longevity Olympics':

Highest healthy life expectancy at birth, both sexes

Country	World ranking
Japan	1
Singapore	2
Spain	3
Switzerland	4
Andorra	5
South Korea	6
Italy	7
Australia	8
Israel	9
Sweden	10
Canada	11
Taiwan	12
France	13

New Zealand	14
Austria	15
Netherlands	16
Germany	17
Costa Rica	18
Ireland	19
Cyprus	20
Malta	21
Greece	22
United Kingdom	23
Chile	24
Portugal	25

Further down the list were the following nations:

Country	World ranking
United States	32
China	34
Kuwait	51
UAE	59
Saudi Arabia	60
North Korea	92
Indonesia	104
Russia	112
Egypt	120
Pakistan	132
India	134
Somalia	175
South Africa	159
Afghanistan	176
Haiti	187 (lowest)

Source: 'Healthy life expectancy [HALE] for 187 countries, 1990–2010: A systematic analysis for the Global Burden Disease Study 2010', *Lancet*, 15 December 2012–4 January 2013. HALE is a snapshot-ranking of projected healthy life expectancy for a child born today, based on current forces of health and mortality.

This book has been researched and written by us both, William and Naomi Moriyama Doyle, but the voice will be Naomi's throughout the book.

The Japanese healthy lifestyle

This is a book about how Japan has discovered, in some ways by accident, a natural, national pattern of eating, moving and thinking that helps its children and adults achieve world-topping healthy longevity rankings, and strikingly better results when compared with a number of other developed nations.

It is an exploration of why children born in Japan, as a national population, are projected to live the longest, healthiest lives on earth – and it's an exploration of possible lessons for parents around the world to help their own children's health and longevity.

I believe that it is a pattern that offers lessons any parent can put into action for their own family, no matter where you live.

In this book I explore why Japanese children are the healthiest on earth and what lessons the rest of the world might learn from them.

Japanese children undoubtedly face many of the challenges that children around the developed world face: excessive screen time, irregular eating patterns, unhealthy fast and 'convenience' foods, counter-productive school and social stress, and less time for free play, relaxation, reading for pleasure and exploring nature. This is not a book that claims that Japanese food or parenting techniques are inherently any better *overall* than those of any other nation. Although very healthy in many respects, Japanese dietary patterns are not perfect, and in some ways they are in the process of a long, gradual shift toward less healthy Western directions. As a nation, Japan in the recent years has been embarking on a nation-wide campaign called *Shokuiku* (Food Education) to reverse the negative trend and bring its population back to more ideal dietary patterns. Nevertheless, experts often rank more traditional Japanese food and lifestyle habits as among the healthiest in the world.

As parents – a Tokyo-born mother and a New York-born father – with a seven-year-old son who is growing up in New York, William and I are new to parenting, and not a day goes by when we don't feel humbled and awed by how much there is to learn, how there are no hard-and-fast formulas for raising children, and how much it is an imperfect, evolutionary process that changes as a family learns, and changes, together.

We are not arguing that children need to eat Japanese food to get healthy, but we have included a collection of Japan-inspired recipes at the end of the book for you to sample and have fun with, if you choose, although they are totally optional.

Finally, this is not a book about emotional, spiritual or other forms of health. The phrase 'World's Healthiest Children' places a somewhat arbitrary focus on physical health, but we feel that physical health and healthy longevity, as estimated by the landmark Global Burden of Disease study published in the *Lancet* in 2012, is a critical reflection of a person's overall health.

The book in a nutshell

The patterns of family thinking, eating and moving that we explore in this book are reflected in the latest recommendations of many of the world's leading experts on children's health and nutrition. These include, for example, the childhood obesity prevention recommendations of the World Health Organization's Global Strategy on Diet, Physical Activity and Health,* which advise:

- Increase consumption of fruit and vegetables, as well as legumes (pulses: peas, beans and lentils), whole grains and nuts.

- Limit energy (calorie) intake from total fats and shift fat consumption away from saturated fats to unsaturated fats.

- Limit the intake of sugars.

- Be physically active – accumulate at least 60 minutes of regular, moderate- to vigorous-intensity activity each day that is developmentally appropriate.

* Note: For guidance on feeding infants and young children see the World Health Organization recommendations in Appendix III, page 201.

These recommendations are simple, but they are often not so easy to put into practice. In writing this book, we have gathered the opinions of a wide variety of leading medical, scientific and academic researchers and experts on child health and nutrition around the world for their insights on helping children lead healthier lives. William and I have also interviewed a fascinating group of women who have interesting insights into children's health and eating habits: a cross-section of Japanese mothers with young children in New York, where many of them were living as expatriates.

From these interviews, seven 'secrets' emerged that I believe can help many parents nurture and improve their child's health, and I will introduce each one in Part 2.

PART 1

How Might We Solve a Worldwide Problem?

1

The Global War on Children's Health

The children of the world are in crisis. Around the globe, the health of our children is under attack, not only from the age-old scourges of infectious disease, hunger, ignorance, war and poverty but also from an onslaught of a relatively new group of enemies created by modern civilisation.

These enemies are childhood obesity, sedentary lifestyles, imbalanced eating habits and the resulting lifestyle-related diseases that can injure our children's health and shorten their lifespan.

Consider these stark realities, reported by the World Health Organization (WHO) and by doctors, scientists and health authorities in the United Kingdom, United States and around the world. According to an analysis published in 2014 in the medical journal *Lancet* using data from the Global Burden of Disease Study, between 1980 and 2013 the worldwide prevalence of overweight and obesity rose by 27.5 per cent for adults and by an even more alarming 47 per cent for children. The study noted that obesity is an issue affecting people of all ages and incomes, everywhere. In 2013, over 22 per cent of girls and boys in developed countries were found to be overweight or obese. 'The rise in obesity among children is especially troubling in so many low and middle-income countries', declared Marie Ng, the paper's lead author. 'We know that there are severe downstream health effects from childhood obesity, including cardiovascular disease, diabetes, and many cancers.'

The health outcomes connected to overweight

According to the WHO, children who are overweight or obese are at greater risk of a range of health problems, including asthma, high blood pressure, musculo-skeletal disorders, fatty liver disease, insulin resistance and type-2 diabetes, as well as obstructive sleep apnoea. In later life, they are at greater risk of obesity, type-2 diabetes, cardiovascular disease, some cancers, obstructive respiratory disease, mental, emotional and social health problems, reproductive disorders and premature death and disability.

'Our perception of what is normal has shifted; being overweight is now more common than unusual,' said WHO official Zsuzsanna Jakab in 2014. 'We must not let another generation grow up with obesity as the new norm. Physical inactivity, coupled with a culture that promotes cheap, convenient foods high in fats, salt and sugars, is deadly.'

So many people are putting on so much weight so quickly that the former chairwoman of the UK's Food Standards Agency, Dame Deirdre Hutton, told *The Times* several years ago, 'When you look at the number of people medically affected by poor diet in terms of ill health or early death from a diet-related disease, we have to do something about it. If you look at the level of obesity in kids and the way it is growing, it's terrifying.'

Our culture seems increasingly engineered to promote obesity. Dr Hermann Toplak of the University of Graz in Austria, and president-elect of the European Association for the Study of Obesity, observed, 'The result is that in today's society many children – and indeed adults – no longer build up enough muscle mass and functionality, and have lost the culture of "classical eating", which has instead been replaced by uncontrolled food intake with a snacking and eating culture.'

The obesity crisis is a worldwide disaster and a public health time bomb. It is spreading into historically lean regions of the Mediterranean and Asia, including Italy, Spain, India and China. Things are getting so bad, that not long ago the Surgeon General of the United States called obesity 'the terror within' and said that unless we do something about it 'the magnitude of the dilemma will dwarf 9/11 or any other terrorist attempt'. Dr Meir Stampfer of the Harvard School of Public Health told WebMD News, 'It is just staggering. This whole epidemic of obesity is sweeping across the country [the US]. One of the difficulties is it's becoming the norm to be overweight. People look down at their bellies, see other people's bellies and see they are average. But in this country, if you are average, you are way overweight.'

In the UK, government data indicates that over 35 per cent of 10- to 11-year-old boys and 32 per cent of girls are overweight, reported the *Guardian* in February 2014. Of those, 20.7 per cent of boys and 17.7 per cent of girls were obese. London cardiologist Dr Aseem Malhotra called obesity 'the greatest threat to health worldwide' and added that 'junk food companies sponsor sporting events and athletes endorse sugary drinks, with advertising that targets the most vulnerable members of society, including children'.

The rise of obesity and diabetes in the UK

Britain has one of the fastest-rising rates of obesity in the developed world, and obesity rates for boys and girls are among the worst in Europe. A recent study ('Prevalence of prediabetes in England from 2003 to 2011', published in *BMJ Open*, June 2014) found that one-third of the population is on the edge of type-2 diabetes, having high blood glucose levels classified as prediabetes. 'If this increase in prediabetes and diabetes isn't tackled now, it will destroy the health service', said Barbara Young, chief executive of Diabetes UK. 'Many of the problems the secretary of state is trying to tackle, such as too many people coming in as emergencies to hospitals, are about the one in six people in any hospital at any time who've got diabetes. So it's a massive impact on the NHS and it's going to get even bigger.'

Ironically, despite the fact that the NHS is the public's primary point of contact for children and family health matters, half of NHS staff are estimated to be obese or overweight. According to an editorial in the December 2014 *Postgraduate Medical Journal* by Dr Malhotra and his colleagues, UK hospitals themselves are awash in cheap, high-calorie, nutrient-poor drinks and snacks. They wrote, 'Confectionary, crisps and sugary drinks are available to staff and patients through vending machines in hospital corridors and to bed-bound patients via hospital trolleys. Also, many hospitals have high-street fast-food franchises on site. Thus acceptability and consumption of such foods is legitimized by being in a healthcare setting.'

According to Dr Kathryn Brown, paediatrician and diabetologist at Gateshead Health NHS Foundation Trust, 'Type-2 diabetes is not just a disease in adults, and over the last two years we have seen an increase in the number of teenagers with the condition. This is mostly related to being severely overweight.' She added, 'It is a huge risk for being on the way to developing complications such as kidney failure and eye problems in early adulthood. It is essential that we get people to be as active as possible and help them eat more healthily if we are to prevent this epidemic getting worse.'

Physical activity has diminished among many societies

In May 2014, *The Times* reported that children in Scotland are among the least active in the world, with the majority of Scottish boys spending over four hours a day playing computer games and watching TV. Additionally, only one in seven Scottish children eat at least five portions of fruit and vegetables a day. Welsh government data reports that rates of childhood obesity in Wales are the highest in the UK, with some 35 per cent of children under 16 years old listed as overweight or obese.

Professor Graham MacGregor, Professor of Cardiovascular Medicine at the Wolfson Institute of Preventive Medicine, Barts and The London School of Medicine and Dentistry, Queen Mary University of London, told us that 'the brilliant advertising that occurs in both the USA and the UK by the food industry (largely managed by previous tobacco executives) makes it very difficult for parents to get their children to eat healthily, and particularly with peer pressure from other children'.

In Ireland, according to University College Dublin lecturer Dr Mimi Tatlow-Golden, 'young children aged three to five years still see upwards of 1,000 TV ads for unhealthy foods over the course of a year'. The UNICEF Report Card 2013 revealed that nearly three-quarters of Irish children aged 11, 13 and 15 spend less than an hour per day engaged in moderate-to-vigorous physical activity. In the 'Growing up in Ireland' report, an estimated 45 per cent of Irish 9-year-olds had a television in their bedrooms, despite the associations identified between TV viewing and poor child health.

A worldwide problem

Obesity is even more of a problem in the US, and some fear that the UK will follow. According to a January 2014 report in the *New England Journal of Medicine* ('Incidence of childhood obesity in the United States'), childhood obesity is a major health problem in the United States. The US Centers for Disease Control report that the percentage of children aged 6–11 years in the United States who were obese increased from 7 per cent in 1980 to nearly 18 per cent in 2012. Similarly, the percentage of adolescents aged 12–19 years who were obese increased from 5 per cent to nearly 21 per cent over the same period.

In a number of developed nations, including the UK, rising childhood obesity rates appear to be levelling off – but they are levelling off at alarmingly high levels. In Australia, for example, according to a January 2010 article in the *International Journal of Obesity* ('Trends in the prevalence of childhood overweight and obesity in Australia between 1985 and 2008') there was a plateau, or only slight increase, in the percentage of boys and girls classified as overweight or obese, with almost no change over the previous 10 years. But the combined prevalence rate for overweight and obesity among Australian boys and girls levelled off at over 25 per cent.

The childhood obesity epidemic is even hitting the Gulf States. The Abu Dhabi Media Company reported in June 2013 that 20 per cent of young people are classified as obese and 14 per cent as overweight.

In China, Western fast-food companies like McDonald's, KFC and Pizza Hut are booming, along with local fast-food chains. At the same time childhood obesity is spiking. McDonald's 1,100 outlets in the country are planned to expand to over 2,000 in the next few years. In July 2014, *China Daily* reported 'an alarming rise in child obesity', with 23 per cent of Chinese young men, and 14 per cent of young women, under 20 estimated to be overweight or obese.

A stunning case history of the children's obesity crisis is unfolding in India, where changing eating habits and a lack of physical activity are taking a terrible toll on young people.

There, children are eating less traditional Indian food and more unhealthy Western food, fast food and processed food, which tends to have more calories, salt and added sugar. Dr Anoop Misra, chairman, Fortis-C-DOC Centre of Excellence for Diabetes, Metabolic Diseases and Endocrinology reported that 'diabesity', or the combination of diabetes and obesity, has become a major problem in India due to lifestyles changes.

> The Indian population is going through a phase of dietary transition. Leaving traditional diets, people have now started opting for packaged foods or quick home-made foods. The increase in the intake of energy [calorie] dense foods, together with low levels of physical activity, are leading to increased obesity and diabetes.

Some Indian experts blame certain aspects of the food culture that encourage the over-feeding of children. As retired paediatrician Dr R.D. Potdar said in the 26 October 2013 issue of the Indian publication *Mid Day*, 'In India, people have a fascination for having chubby babies. So from early childhood itself, parents feed their baby with the aim of making them fat. Now, kids get used to street food and junk food from school itself. They put on weight easily.'

Dr Shashank Shah, a bariatric and laparoscopic surgeon, noticed 'a lack of awareness among parents'. He also told *Mid Day*:

Parents often take their kids out for pizzas and junk food. With the intake of junk food, there is hardly any ground sport. Kids are always on the computer and playing video games. The open spaces are vanishing so fast, there is hardly any space for kids to play, these days. I have come across so many cases of young people who are already suffering from obesity or are overweight, suffering from diabetes by the age of 25. Eventually by the age of 40, they have serious heart problems.

'With time, even children below two years are getting hooked on television,' said paediatrician Dr Pallab Chatterjee in an interview with the *Hindustan Times*. 'According to internationally accepted guidelines, this is not a normal routine. For children above two years, watching TV should be restricted to maximum two hours [per day].' According to Arpita Adhikary, lifestyle counsellor at Apollo Hospital, children are 'staying glued' to electronic gadgets like laptops and tablets, 'and as these children grow up, they become unwilling to go out' and play in the real world.

In the UK, the Institute of Economic Affairs, a free market think tank, published a contrarian report in 2014 titled 'The Fat Lie'. The paper used data from the Department for Environment, Food and Rural Affairs (DEFRA) to argue that 'per capita consumption of sugar, salt, fat and calories has been falling in Britain for decades' and that the rise in obesity has mainly been triggered 'by a decline in physical activity at home and in the workplace, not an increase in sugar, fat or calorie consumption'. Critics of the report pointed out that the DEFRA data is based on 'self-reporting' by consumers surveyed, which can be highly inaccurate and misleading, but regardless, declining physical activity is probably a critical factor adding to the obesity crisis, for both adults and children.

What are the causes?

Why are so many children around the world suffering from obesity, poor diets and physical inactivity?

The problem, it seems, is due to a major imbalance in the quality and quantity of the food we eat and the way that imbalance interacts with our lifestyle in an increasingly obesogenic, or obesity-promoting, society. According to the theories of experts who have studied the problem of obesity and children's health, our children and families are:

- Eating more calories than we burn off, or falling into a calorie imbalance.

- Not getting enough physical activity and becoming more sedentary in our daily lives; for example, watching more TV and spending leisure time with electronic devices instead of being physically active.

- Eating more super-sized fast-food meals.

- Eating portion sizes that often have expanded in size over the past decades.

- Eating more junk food and snacks.

- Eating more unhealthy takeaways and ready meals.

- Eating more processed food, and less complex carbohydrates and dietary fibre.

- Being over-exposed to the wrong nutritional choices at schools and social situations.

- Drinking too many sweetened fizzy drinks.

- Losing the skills, time or desire to make healthier meals for ourselves and our families.

- Feeding infants and children too much calorie-dense, high-fat, high-sugar and high-salt foods.

- The aggressive marketing of 'calorie-dense, nutrient-poor' foods and beverages to children and families further exacerbates the problem.

- In some societies, longstanding cultural norms, like the common belief that a fat baby is a healthy baby, may encourage families to over-feed their children.

- The increasingly urbanised and digitalised world offers fewer opportunities for physical activity through healthy play. Being overweight or obese further reduces children's opportunities to participate in group physical activities. They then become even less physically active, which makes them likely to become more overweight over time.

Childhood obesity seems to be an exquisitely complex problem, with biological, cultural and psychological roots that are difficult to trace and disentangle. As researchers Joan C. Han, Debbie A. Lawlor and Sue Y.S. Kimm pointed out in a May 2010 report in the *Lancet* ('Childhood obesity – 2010: Progress and challenges'), about 50 years ago, a huge shift occurred: at the same time the food supply stabilised in developed nations with an abundance of cheap, high-calorie foods, the amount of regular physical activity needed for daily life dropped off sharply, creating a huge imbalance in 'calories in/calories out'. The result: an epidemic of obesity.

As it happens, though, there is one nation in the world that has both captured the number-one position in the world ranking of healthy longevity and held the line on childhood obesity to a very low level relative to the rest of the world. That country is Japan.

2

Why are Japanese Children the Healthiest on Earth?

Sleep, sleep, sleep, little one,
While my baby sleeps I will wash some red beans, and
*   clean some rice, Then*
adding some fish to the red rice,
I will serve it up to this best of little babies.

Japanese lullaby

What do the Japanese do differently? What is it that Japanese children do in their daily life that helps them enjoy the world's longest healthy lives and relatively low levels of obesity, and how might our children living in other nations benefit from those lessons? To find the possible answers, William and I interviewed doctors, researchers, scientists and public-health experts in Japan and around the world. We travelled with our young son to Tokyo and deep into the Japanese countryside to my father's ancestral home, which is still a working farm managed by my cousins and their families.

We looked for answers in Japanese homes, schools, research institutions, supermarkets and farmers' markets. We asked for the opinions and insights of Japanese mothers, fathers and grandparents, and nursery and kindergarten teachers and school nutritionists. And we gradually discovered that there is a series of cultural factors and essential life-changing behaviours exhibited by Japanese children that, taken together, according to the best expert opinions, may give them a decisive healthy-longevity advantage over the rest of the world.

The healthy rhythm of life in Japan

In short, overall, not only do Japanese children live in a developed nation with a highly advanced health-care system, but they also enjoy a healthier food pattern and habits, a daily rhythm of life that leads them to enjoy a high level of physical activity (in a way you might not expect) and a culture that supports children's healthy-lifestyle behaviours.

I also came to realise that there are seven fundamental research-based 'secrets' that I will be describing in Part 2, that may help children and parents in any part of the world enjoy some of the same advantages that Japanese children do.

As William and I conducted our family journey, a host of long-forgotten memories came back to me of my own childhood in Japan, and of sitting at the dinner table with my family and extended family.

When my son was born, my parents flew over from Tokyo to New York to meet him. On their first night in New York, my mother, Chizuko, whipped up a Japanese-style home-cooked meal in our kitchen from local American ingredients she found in the supermarket, and my dad, Shigeo, rocked his new grandson in his arms. Before long, as the kitchen filled with the aromas of authentic, super-healthy Japanese-style home cooking – made from easily available local New York ingredients – you could hear the sounds of old-fashioned Japanese lullabies and folk songs being sung by a new grandmother and grandfather to a three-month-old baby.

Like mothers everywhere, Japanese mums show their love for their children through healthy, delicious food. And through a combination of natural wisdom and the accidents of history and geography, Japanese parents have happened on a rhythm of lifestyle behaviours, food choices and recipes that have helped create the healthiest children on earth, and a nation of 'little foodies', or children who instinctively gravitate toward a very healthy overall eating pattern.

Adapting the Japanese approach in other countries

When I became a mother myself seven years ago, I was determined to help my son enjoy really healthy eating patterns, through the most nutritious and delicious foods. Some days it works out, like the day he ate his first solid food – mashed avocado – and the many times he enjoyed his favourite snacks of steamed sweet potatoes and sautéed beetroot, and the many mornings when my American husband serves the family an old-school Japanese breakfast. (Confession: he takes lots of shortcuts, so it only takes about five minutes.)

Then, on other days, it seems like wall-to-wall 'kids menus' – featuring pizza, cupcakes, crisps and French fries – in the same way that it does for many families. Still, as a family, we try, and often succeed, in staying focused on healthy eating overall, by adapting and adopting the wisdom of the land where I was born.

The goodness and wisdom of Japanese-style eating and other healthy traditional eating patterns lies all around us, however, in the choices you can make every day at your supermarkets, grocers, farmers' markets and restaurants. You can make it happen right in your own kitchen and dining room, without necessarily ever having to learn how to prepare the kind of food you eat in a Japanese restaurant.

This book is a celebration of healthy living and delicious food for children, based on the best scientific insights. It is an exploration of how Japanese people approach their children's food and lifestyles, and how they have discovered some great natural wisdom along the way.

It is a treasury of Japanese-style recipes for you and your children to enjoy and have fun with, and to work into your family's own healthy-eating pattern.

Rediscovering the wisdom of Japan

When our son was three years old, he was fascinated with Japanese 'bullet trains', or *shinkansen*, and he dreamed about them constantly.

At the same time, I dreamed of showing him the world where I grew up, and I wanted to work out how I could build a simple daily system of three meals and healthy snacks for him when we got back to the United States – and make it as simple as possible. When my son was four years old, he and I boarded a flight from New York to Tokyo – the 'old country' – and we lived as local Japanese for the summer.

As the journey unfolded, I began to discover the Japanese mother inside me, and wished to return to America with as much wisdom I could, to help my son live a healthy life through the right food choices for meals and snacks, plus allowances for indulgence, sweets, fun and even a little decadence, Japanese-style. And I wished to share the wisdom, and distil it into simple, easy-to-follow insights, so that other parents might benefit.

We marvelled at the ultra-premium gourmet food courts at upmarket department stores, shopped at the local Tokyo supermarkets, and helped my mother prepare super-healthy everyday Japanese-style meals. We took a *shinkansen* bullet train past Mount Fuji into the Japanese countryside, and we stayed at my family's working country farm in the little rural mountain hamlet of Kozaka. There, I relived my childhood memories, picking fresh tangerines from the trees and being immersed in Japanese food culture and seasonal food festivals and events.

It seemed that everywhere we went, we saw many healthy-looking children, in a nation that is far from perfect, but where young people are blessed, without necessarily even knowing it, with a lifestyle, culture and dietary pattern that is one of the healthiest on earth.

What is the secret behind the health of the Japanese?

Why will children born in Japan today enjoy the longest, healthiest lives on earth?

The short answer is that researchers aren't exactly sure – but they have some pretty good ideas. You might think that Japanese people have a decisive genetic advantage for longevity, but research has refuted this idea. As cardiologist Dr Robert Vogel of University of Maryland School of Medicine told us for our previous book, *The Japan Diet*, 'You might think it's in the genes, but it looks like genes don't help much. We know from the NiHonSan [Nippon-Japan, Honolulu, San Francisco] study that Japanese genes play little, if any, role in their longevity, since Japanese moving to Honolulu or San Francisco develop the same heart disease rates and longevity as do locals.' Dr Michel de Lorgeril, Chief Scientist Investigator at the French National Centre for Scientific Research, leader of the Lyons Diet Heart Study and a leading expert on the French and Mediterranean diets agrees, telling us, 'Studies have shown that Japanese are not protected [from disease] by their genes.'

One probable reason for Japan's longevity edge versus the rest of the world is its culture of health – its free universal health coverage and world-class medical system, and its cultural stress on cleanliness and hygiene. Japan has sharply cut infectious disease and infant mortality rates, reduced its high death rate from stroke with salt-reduction campaigns and blood pressure drugs; and encourages mass health screenings in school and regular check-ups that are so comprehensive they're called 'human drydocks'. Other probable factors include Japan's very strong ties of community and friends, a national sense of *ikigai*, or purpose of life, and a culture of stress reduction through contemplative pursuits.

The leading Japanese researcher for the *Lancet* study, Professor Kenji Shibuya and his colleagues at the department of global health policy at the University of Tokyo, identified three possible critical factors, including the Japanese dietary pattern, that may explain Japanese longevity:

Japanese people give attention to hygiene in all aspects of their daily life. This attitude might partly be attributable to a complex interaction of culture, education, climate, environment and the Shinto tradition of purifying the body and mind before meeting others. Second, they are health conscious. In Japan regular check-ups are the norm. Mass screening is provided for everyone at school and work or in the community by local government authorities. Third, Japanese food has a balanced nutritional benefit and the diet of the population has improved in tandem with economic development.

'Japan: Universal Health Care at 50 Years',
Lancet, 30 August 2011

The 12 life-changing behaviours of Japanese children

There are at least 12 interconnected lifestyle factors that are also possible contributors to the Japanese healthy-longevity edge. When compared to children in other developed countries, on average, Japanese children:

1 Enjoy a national food pattern that is relatively higher in nutrients, is more efficiently filling by likely being lower in calorie density or 'calories per bite', and which features higher proportions of fish and plant-based foods, with a lower proportion of meat and fewer total calories.

2 Are inspired from infancy to try to enjoy a wider variety of different healthy foods, including many different fruits and vegetables.

3 Are served food on smaller plates, with little super-sizing.

4 Are taught to practise flexible restraint, not severe food restriction or food demonisation.

5 Are encouraged to enjoy treats and snacks, but in the right amounts and frequency.

6 Have large amounts of routine physical activity, or 'incidental exercise', built into their daily lives.

7 Are given 'smart rewards' for regular exercise.

8 Often eat meals together with their family as a regular ritual, with at least one parent (often the mother) present throughout the meal.

9 Have 'wrap-around' home and school environments that support healthier food and lifestyle choices.

10 Are supported by parents who model and educate healthy eating for them, and require that schools do the same.

11 Are supported by parents who communicate food and lifestyle wisdom in an authori*tative* rather than authori*tarian* style.

12 Are taught from early childhood to be chef's assistants, food servers and cleaner-uppers.

The result, when compared with the rest of the world, is nothing less than a public-health miracle.

Although childhood obesity among children in a number of developed nations is growing at alarmingly high levels – or evening out, as seems to be the case in the UK – and a raging obesity epidemic is engulfing millions of children the world over, Japanese childhood obesity levels have historically been much lower, and have in fact been declining overall in recent years. There are eating disorders among young women in Japan, such as anorexia and excessive thinness, but they are at levels that are lower, for example, than in the US.

In fact, Japan, along with South Korea, has held the line against childhood obesity most effectively among the developed nations. This probably provides a major advantage for healthy longevity, since lifelong eating patterns are often established in childhood.

Japan again tops the world at number 1

	Childhood obesity only	Childhood obesity and overweight
Japan	2.9	13.9
South Korea	4.0	17.1
Sweden	4.2	19.6
Norway	4.6	18.0
China	4.9	18.5
France	5.2	18.1
Germany	5.2	20.1
Taiwan	5.6	21.1
Switzerland	6.0	18.4
Poland	6.4	19.8
Australia	7.1	23.7
Ireland	7.1	26.7
Russia	7.3	20.5
Italy	7.3	26.9
Denmark	7.4	19.5
UK	7.7	27.5
Finland	7.8	23.3
Spain	8.1	25.8
Austria	9.0	17.5
Greece	9.2	31.3
Canada	9.4	23.8
New Zealand	9.5	29.2
Saudi Arabia	12.0	30.0
Israel	12.7	29.0
United States	13.0	29.5
Kuwait	17.7	34.8

2013 obesity prevalence (per cent) for children aged 2–19, both sexes, for select countries.

Source: Institute for Health Metrics and Evaluation, University of Washington
http://healthmetricsandevaluation.org
http://vizhub.healthdata.org/obesity/

What's more, it turns out that the Japanese lifestyle – the way Japanese people eat, move and think – may also be critical in establishing Japan's number-one position in healthy longevity and in low childhood obesity.

The 12 lifestyle patterns described on pages 17–18 can be grouped into a series of just seven simple, breakthrough, Japan-inspired, expert-approved insights that form the core of this book, and I hope you will consider applying these to your own family. These insights I call 'seven secrets to nurture your child's health'.

PART 2

The Seven Secrets to Nurture Your Child's Health

Tweak Your Family Meals to Make Them Nutrient-dense

Enjoy family meals that are higher in nutrients, include
more plant-based foods and whole grains, and contain
less processed food, added sugars and salt.

Eating local vegetables will strengthen health.

Japanese saying

You don't have to eat Japanese food to help nurture one of the
world's healthiest children – just give your family's food habits a
Japanese-style tweak.

When I was growing up in Japan, a common meal at our
house, and many other Japanese homes, was a bowl of miso soup,
a glass of water or barley tea, a bowl of plain short-grain rice, a
small piece of fish or tofu, and two or three veggie-based side
dishes, finished off with a piece of fruit.

We didn't realise it at the time, but my mother had been
feeding us her version of the traditional Japanese diet, a style of
healthy eating that, along with other traditional eating patterns
around the world, like the Mediterranean diet, can be considered
a gold standard of healthy eating.

As late as the 1950s and 1960s, many British children may
have also had a healthier diet, in part because it was also more

'traditional': fewer processed foods, more home-cooked meals, and fewer empty calories when compared with today, combined with more routine physical activity.

My mother still serves meals that way. Like many mothers and grandmothers around the world, my mother has stayed connected to a highly nutritious, traditional healthy dietary pattern. It is an organic process that she follows, not because it's on the cutting edge of nutritional science, but because it naturally feels like the right thing to do.

At almost the exact moment in history that I returned to Tokyo for several years after attending college in the US, the Japanese nation was enjoying a fleeting golden age of 'nutritional balance'. The government of Japan considers the year 1980 as the point in time when the national diet was in a state of 'balance' between Eastern and Western food styles and calorie content, and with a healthy balance of food types eaten.

Japan's food culture has undeniably become more Westernised and globalised over the years, and in some ways not for the better. But today, Japanese adults and children enjoy a national diet that is, when compared with other developed nations, still relatively lower in calories, higher in nutrients, more efficiently filling by being lower in calorie density or 'calories per bite', and it features more fish and plant-based foods, with less meat and added sugars.

Many experts place the Japanese diet on a par with the fabled traditional Mediterranean diet. When combined with excellent food education in Japanese schools, the happy result of this diet is that, according to Takuya Mitani, health education official with Japan's Education Ministry, after a modest spike in childhood obesity at the turn of the century, 'Obesity rates have been gradually decreasing since 2003 in children and teens' in Japan.

The ultimate family meal foundation

What would be the perfect eating pattern to achieve the healthiest, longest life? The experts don't really know for sure, since long-term randomised trial studies of different diets on human beings, the hypothetical 'gold standard' in such research, are rarely even attempted, since it's nearly impossible to get people to adhere to a specific diet for 5, 10 or 20 years. Assistant Professor Christopher Gardner, of the University of Stanford School of Medicine, told me, 'What we should do is randomly assign 100,000 people to eat a lot of soy, or not, and follow them for 100 years and see who lives longer. And that's never going to happen.' So what we're stuck with, said Gardner, are imperfect studies with significant limitations. 'You'll never get the perfect studies,' he concluded, 'so what you do is piece together the different parts of the puzzle.'

Around the globe, however, many of the world's best experts are starting to believe that there may be a unified theory of health and nutrition that can help minimise the risks of obesity and the hosts of illnesses it triggers, and maximise the probability of a long, healthy life.

The emerging theory, which validates the wisdom of Japanese and other traditional healthy-eating patterns, is based in part on the pioneering work of Prof. Barbara Rolls and her team of researchers at the University of Pennsylvania. They have conducted a series of studies indicating that a dietary pattern of foods high in fibre and water content like fruit and vegetables, and low in calorie density – or 'calories per bite' – has an extraordinary double benefit: it protects against overeating and obesity, and it delivers a package of nutrients that can maximise health and possibly longevity. Japan, as it turns out, is a relative 'low-calorie-density Utopia'. Japanese-style eating is very efficient in both filling power and in delivering a high-quality nutrient package.

One secret: Japan's default meal foundation is rice, much more than bread or other forms of processed wheat, which is very different to Western diets. The advantage of Japanese-style short-grain rice, preferably brown, or the incredibly good-tasting *haiga* partially milled rice (you can get it at an Asian market or online), is that it is water-rich when cooked, fluffy and super-filling and much lower in calorie density than bread.

All that belly-filling rice might also displace less healthy foods and reduce the overall number of calories eaten. According to United Nations Food and Agriculture Organization estimates, the calorie availability per person in Japan is roughly 2,700 calories per day, vs 3,400 for the UK and 3,600 a day for the US. And overall, the Japanese food pattern, or the general combination of specific foods, is believed by many experts to be healthier than more 'Western' patterns.

For parents, the challenge is how to guide children into such a pattern early on, and this is where the secrets of the world's healthiest children come in. For generations, Japanese parents have known instinctively that a (mostly) full belly is a happy belly and, as the Japanese saying suggests, *hara hache bun me*, or 'eat until you're 80 per cent full'. In other words, the objective of eating is not to quickly stuff yourself but to gradually allow yourself to be satisfied.

The most intriguing point: Japanese people eat many of the same basic types of foods as people in the UK or US, but what's different is the quantity, the balance and the variety of food.

A changing diet

Although the Japanese national diet is becoming more and more Westernised, and there are plenty of unhealthy food choices on sale in Japan, Japanese people today still eat dramatically more fish, belly-filling veggies and rice, and dramatically less added sugar, meat and overall calories than, for example, people in the UK. When combined with high levels of what is called 'incidental exercise' or routine physical activity, the overall symphony of Japanese eating patterns may give Japanese people a critical advantage for healthy weight and longevity.

Prof. Frank Hu of the Harvard University School of Public Health told me, 'Plant-based diets like the Japanese or Asian diets are a combination of high consumption of vegetables, fruits, grain products including rice and also a high consumption of seafood. A dietary pattern higher in fruits, vegetables, whole grains and fish/seafood has been consistently associated with a lower risk of chronic diseases. These kinds of plant-based foods certainly have had a lot of scientific support in the past several decades in terms of their benefits on cardiovascular disease, cancer prevention and also longevity.'

While childhood obesity levels among many children in the UK appear to be levelling off at high levels, and a raging obesity epidemic is engulfing millions of children the world over, Japanese childhood obesity levels have historically been much lower. Of course, as we have seen, there are eating problems and disorders in Japan, but such disorders exist at lower levels than in, for example, the US. In fact, Japan has held the line against childhood obesity more effectively than any other developed nation, which is another advantage for healthy longevity, since lifelong eating patterns are often established in childhood.

Salt

Admittedly, there is too much sodium in the Japanese diet, in foods such as salted dried fish, and pickled vegetables, and from what I consider as the overuse of soy sauce. Japanese men also smoke at an alarmingly high rate and alcohol-related ailments are also high. But Japanese obesity is the lowest in the developing world, in part because of a tradition of smaller portions than in the West, and a somewhat different food culture.

The contrast between UK, US and Japanese diets

For a snapshot of how Japanese food patterns stack up against those in the UK, and those in the US, an example of the direction you don't want to go in, have a look at these recent figures from the United Nations Food and Agriculture Organization. Note that this is not precise consumption data, but estimates of total per capita daily calories, including waste and spoilage. While the numbers are somewhat rough, they are broadly reflective of national food patterns:

What the Japanese do differently – the national food pattern

	Japan	UK	US
Total daily calories available	2,719	3,414	3,639
Percentage of total calories:			
As vegetable products	80%	71%	73%
As animal products	20%	29%	27%
A few key items, percentage of total calories			
Rice	21%	2%	2%
Fish and seafood	5%	1%	1%
Total meat	7%	13%	12%

Source: 2011 FAO Balance Sheets, food supply in kcal, per person, per day.

Japanese food patterns are based on a total daily calorie availability of about 2,700 calories per person, or about 700 less than the UK and 1,000 less than in the US.

The Japanese national food pattern appears to be more 'calorie-corrected' than the UK diet – it is closer to the ideal roughly 2,000 to 2,800 calories many adults need to maintain a healthy weight, a number which depends on gender, activity levels and body type.

Since the pattern of foods eaten in Japan is probably lower in calorie density, which means lower in calories per bite and higher in belly-filling water content in the form of vegetables, fruit and rice, those 2,700 available calories are more efficient at being filling and satisfying than the typical UK or US pattern.

In contrast to children in the UK, US and many parts of Europe, Japanese children are growing up in a nation where less-healthy and higher-calorie eating patterns are less common. This helps Japanese children maintain a relatively healthy weight over time, and avoid the health risks of obesity.

Japanese dietary patterns are based on more vegetable products as a percentage of total calories. This includes water-rich, belly-filling rice, a staple of many Asian diets. These figures do not fully break down which individual vegetable products add up to the totals, but my strong anecdotal impression is that Japanese people are, from childhood, inspired to eat a wider range of healthy fruit and vegetables from the land and sea than other developed nations.

An emphasis on vegetables and fruit

Nutritional authorities around the world are telling us of the health benefits of eating a wide variety of fruits and vegetables, preferably in their whole form without added sugar or deep-fat frying. This simple, straightforward global insight is as old as our grandparents' and parents' wisdom and as new as today's cutting-edge clinical research: if you want to help maximise your health and fight chronic illness, eat a diet that is rich in many different fruits and vegetables.

Even today, after decades of Westernisation, vegetables still occupy a major portion of the Japanese diet. Plant-based products are a higher proportion of the Japanese diet compared with the UK and US, and Japanese people may eat a wider variety of veggies. Japanese cuisine puts vegetables at the centre of a meal, transforming many different kinds of seasonal veggies into a series of colourful dishes bursting with flavours. You'd be amazed at the wide range of ways that vegetables are prepared in Japan: steamed, sautéed with subtle seasonings, simmered in delicious broth, dressed in a mild vinaigrette, or dressed in a miso-based barbecue-like sauce. (See the recipes at the end of the book for some examples.)

How can vegetables and fruit help protect your family's health?

Vegetables and fruit can help you feel full on fewer calories, according to a widely respected theory of diet and nutrition called 'energy density' or 'calorie density'. This theory has been popularised by Dr Barbara Rolls, chair of the nutrition department at Penn State University. According to Dr Rolls, 'Fruits and vegetables really are key players in determining weight status.' The calorie-density theory says that if you eat more low-calorie-dense foods and fewer high-calorie-dense foods, you will more effectively reach satiety, or fullness, and eat fewer calories overall. Low-calorie-dense foods and dishes include fruit, vegetables, low-fat milk, cooked grains, lean meat, poultry, fish, beans, broth-based soups, stews, pasta with vegetables and fruit-based desserts. High-calorie-dense foods include foods like crackers, crisps, chocolate, sweets and biscuits.

The secret ingredient, according to this approach, is water, which dilutes the amount of calories in a given portion of food. 'Surprisingly, foods with a high water content have a big (positive) impact on satiety', wrote Dr Rolls. Of fruit and vegetables, she wrote: 'These carbohydrate-containing [plant-based] foods are truly extraordinary. You can eat virtually as much as you want of many of these and you'll wind up consuming fewer calories.' Here's the mysterious thing about fruit and vegetables: we know that they contain health-promoting substances, but we don't yet know much about how they work. 'Many people who know a little about phytochemicals [plant compounds that can support health] are waiting to hear about the one compound which, taken in large doses, will cure whatever ails them,' explained registered dietician Karen Collins. 'Is it lycopene, beta-carotene, or res-veratrol? In fact, research seems to indicate that phytochemicals work together to boost our immune system. So you benefit by eating a great variety of plant foods containing a great variety of phytochemicals.'

In other words, the beneficial substances in fruit and vegetables seem to work in teams and highly complex patterns, so we shouldn't get too caught up in a single phytochemical or a list of only 'top 10 super-vegetables'. 'It is likely', wrote epidemiologist Dr Lyn Steffen of the University of Minnesota School of Public

Health, in the January 2006 issue of the *Lancet*, 'that the combination of nutrients and compounds in foods has greater health benefits than the individual nutrient alone.' The bottom line is that we need to eat a variety of fruit and vegetables to make sure we get all the nutrients we need.

One day on the campus of Stanford University Medical School in California, a nutritional scientist, Christopher Gardner, took time off from his research to talk about a tasty subject, and one of his favourite dishes, stir-fried vegetables. Gardner specialises in the role of nutrition and preventive medicine. He has published papers on soya and garlic, plant-based diets and phytochemicals, and cardiovascular disease and cancer prevention. But when you hear the passion in Gardner's voice when he speaks of cooking and ingredients and colours and flavours, you get the feeling that perhaps he's really in the business as much for the food as for the science.

He told me:

If you look at the Japanese diet, the Mediterranean diet or the DASH [Dietary Approaches to Stop Hypertension] diet, there's a common theme: they are plant-based and nutrient-dense. Look at what Asians put into their stir-fries. The typical Japanese meal is *flavoured* with strips of fish or chicken or beef. It's not a 12-ounce porterhouse steak. There's rice, herbs that make it smell great and taste great, they've got water chestnuts and mangetouts and mung sprouts, pak choi, mustard greens, just a wonderful variety of colours and flavours. If you add it up, there are the classic vitamins, nutrients, phytochemicals and isoflavones. It's not just what you should avoid, it's what you should include in your diet. You should include the nutrient-dense foods, of which you will find a lot in the Japanese diet. They're in vegetables, they're in beans, they're in whole grains. If you look at the emerging [scientific] literature, these positive factors always seem to be coming, or at least 99 per cent of them, from the plant-based sources.

Veggie variety is the key

According to experts at institutions such as the Harvard University School of Public Health and the US Centers for Disease Control, eating lots of different vegetables and fruits – including dark leafy greens, tomatoes, berries, citrus fruits, sweet potatoes, beans, and fruit and vegetables of all colours and types – may help ward off heart disease and stroke, control blood pressure, prevent some types of cancer, protect against obesity and type-2 diabetes, and protect against cataract and macular degeneration, two common causes of vision loss. The bottom line, according to the Harvard University School of Public Health: 'Vegetables and fruits are clearly an important part of a good diet. Almost everyone can benefit from eating more of them, but variety is as important as quantity. No single fruit or vegetable provides all of the nutrients you need to be healthy. The key lies in the variety of different vegetables and fruits that you eat.'

Think patterns more than superfoods

Among many experts, the once-popular idea of a list of elite superfoods is now giving way to the idea that the real superfood is an eating pattern based on a foundation of a wide variety of different vegetables and fruits, including pulses such as beans and peas. According to the US Centers for Disease Control (CDC), fruits and vegetables are sources of many vitamins, minerals and other natural substances that can help to protect us from chronic diseases. Eating a pattern of foods that includes a wide variety of fruits and vegetables of different colours gives your body a wide range of valuable nutrients, such as fibre, folate, potassium and vitamins A and C, to name just a few.

By one estimate, the Japanese eat an average of up to an astonishing 100 different kinds of food per week (versus Americans at only 30, and Europeans at 45), but still manage to consume over 20 per cent fewer calories than Americans.

The health power of fruit and vegetables

Here, according to the CDC, are just a few examples of the health benefits of eating family meals that have a variety of fruits and vegetables as their foundation:

Fibre Diets rich in dietary fibre have been shown to have a number of beneficial effects, including decreased risk of coronary artery disease.
Excellent vegetable sources: haricot beans, kidney beans, black beans, pinto beans, butter beans, cannellini beans, soya beans, split peas, chickpeas, black-eyed peas, lentils, artichokes.

Folate* Healthy diets with adequate folate might reduce a woman's risk of having a child with a brain or spinal cord defect. For everyone else, folate and folic acid help many healthy body functions, including the production of DNA.
Excellent vegetable sources: black-eyed peas, cooked spinach, haricot beans, asparagus.

Potassium Diets rich in potassium might help to maintain a healthy blood pressure.
Excellent fruit and vegetable sources: sweet potatoes, tomato purée, beetroot greens, potatoes, cannellini beans, butter beans, cooked greens, carrot juice, prune juice.

Vitamin A keeps the eyes and skin healthy and helps to protect against infections.
Excellent fruit and vegetable sources: sweet potatoes, pumpkin, carrots, spinach, turnip greens, mustard greens, kale, spring greens, butternut squash and other autumn squashes, cantaloupe melon, red peppers, Chinese cabbage.

---

* The Institute of Medicine recommends that women of childbearing age who may become pregnant consume 400mcg (micrograms) of synthetic folic acid per day to supplement the folate they receive from a varied diet. Synthetic folic acid can be obtained from eating fortified foods or taking a supplement

Vitamin C helps to heal cuts and wounds and keeps teeth and gums healthy.

EXCELLENT FRUIT AND VEGETABLE SOURCES: red and green peppers, kiwi fruit, strawberries, sweet potatoes, kale, cantaloupe melon, broccoli, pineapple, Brussels sprouts, oranges, mangoes, tomato juice, cauliflower.

Fish – an exceptional food

Japanese dietary patterns are based on more of the good fats from fish, and less meat. The abundance of fish in the Japanese diet may have two benefits compared to more Western patterns: it reduces the volume of saturated fat contained in meat, which is believed to be a possible contributor to certain health risks if eaten in excessively high amounts and frequencies, and the unsaturated omega-3 fatty acids in fish, especially oily fish, may offer protection against certain forms of heart disease.

In our previous book, *The Japan Diet*, we wrote about a man in Pennsylvania who has uncovered a mystery about Japan. 'There's something about the Japanese diet and lifestyle that seems to be unique,' he said, and it may help protect Japanese people against coronary heart disease, one of the world's biggest killers.

It is a paradox, something he can't exactly work out, but he has an interesting theory and it involves the power of fish. Dr Lewis Kuller is an elder statesman in the field of epidemiology, the study of populations and public health. He has studied medicine for nearly 50 years, he is a doctor of medicine and Professor of Public Health at the University of Pittsburgh Graduate School of Public Health. He has published over 500 articles in medical journals. Kuller and his colleagues in Japan have been studying patterns of diet and disease among Japanese people and comparing them to populations elsewhere in the world. And they've noticed something that he finds absolutely fascinating.

According to Dr Kuller, among older Japanese men, there has been a shift towards more Western lifestyles and eating habits. They are eating more saturated fat, meat and cheese than their elders did. They are very heavy smokers. They have hypertension and they are becoming less physically active.

Dr Kuller reasons that we should be seeing a sharp increase in coronary heart disease among Japanese (especially men) and there should be an epidemic of heart attacks in Japan. In fact, thinks Kuller, you'd expect the rates to be going 'off the scale'. But they're not. Dr Kuller reports: 'There's very little evidence of an increase in coronary heart disease incidence or mortality in the Japanese population, especially in the fairly young Japanese population. That to me is an important unexplained paradox.'

It's not a genetic effect unique to Asians, Dr Kuller reasons, because 'we've studied the Japanese in America, Brazil and Hawaii, and their rates are much higher' than those in Japan. Also, the Chinese are seeing increasing rates of coronary heart disease, and rates are going up in Taiwan, South Korea and Singapore as well. 'It may well be that something in the [Japanese] diet is protective, which we could add to our diet,' he speculates. He can't prove it, but if he had to place a bet today, Kuller said he'd wager that the answer to the paradox is that the Japanese enjoy 'an extraordinarily high intake of omega-3 fatty acids from fish'.

Lots of fish means lots of healthy omega-3 fats

The Japan I grew up in was truly a fish-crazed nation and it still is today. The food culture is intensely focused on celebrating fish in the daily diet, in an enormous range of varieties and cooking styles. The Japanese are fish-eating champions of the world, not only beating the UK and the US by a wide margin, but, according to Dr Kuller, 'they eat a lot more fish than the Chinese' and 'about twice as much as the Koreans'.

Kuller's theory is that it's the very high intake of omega-3s in the Japanese diet that is heart-protective and a key factor contributing towards the high longevity of the Japanese people.

What does it mean for us in the West? 'Keeping saturated fat as low as possible and dramatically increasing the amount of omega-3 fatty acids in the diet might have very big benefits,' said Kuller, 'and we need to find that out.'

As with so much in the diet and nutrition world, the research on fish is not iron clad. Many studies have suggested various health benefits for fatty fish, mainly in protecting the heart. But a 2006 review paper in the *British Medical Journal* found little firm evidence of such benefits, leading Joe Schwarcz, Professor of Chemistry at McGill University, to write that 'it is clear that we cannot swallow all the hype about the supposed miraculous properties of omega-3 fats hook, line and sinker'. He speculated, 'Maybe the benefits of fish are not in what they contain, but in what they displace from the diet.'

If Dr Kuller is right about the benefits that Japanese people enjoy from fish, his theory would dovetail with a consensus that is emerging throughout the nutritional world: the right kinds of fat are beneficial to health. More specifically, good fats, or unsaturated fats such as the omega-3s in fish, can be an important component of a healthy diet.

Fish and safety

There has been controversy and some confusion about the safety of fish, owing to fears over contaminants that some species may contain, such as mercury and polychlorinated biphenyls (PCBs: industrial by-products, now banned, that still persist in the environment). The most problematic fish are long-lived predatory species, such as marlin, shark and swordfish. They are at the top of the food chain and so may accumulate large amounts of contaminants from the fish they prey on. Some researchers have also raised concerns over what they see as high levels of PCBs found in farmed salmon, from the fish oil and fish meal they are fed on. But the advantages of eating fish 'are likely to be at least 100-fold greater than the estimates of harm, which may not exist at all', argued Walter Willett, Professor of Nutrition at the Harvard School of Public Health.

How to ramp up your family's omega-3s

- Canned Alaskan salmon, herring, mackerel and sardines are fabulous ways to enjoy omega-3-rich oily fish regularly, and you can eat them straight out of the can. They are super-convenient and they are as nutritious as fresh. The skin and soft bones in canned salmon are completely edible and good for you, too. Look for canned fish with less added salt.
- Instead of fried fish, choose healthier options like poached, baked, steamed or grilled fish.
- A good plant-based source of omega-3 fatty acids is flaxseed (though probably not quite as good as fish), which is available in many supermarkets and health-food shops. It has a light, nutty taste and you can sprinkle it into cereal, soups and many other foods. To unlock the power of the omega-3s, it's best to buy ground flaxseed, or you can grind the seeds yourself.

Flavour bursts for fish

Instead of serving fish with mayonnaise, tartar sauce, hollandaise sauce or butter, try seasoning it with lemon juice or chopped herbs. Traditional Japanese-style flavourings include a small mound of grated radish, such as daikon (also called mooli), and a few drops of lower-salt soy sauce; or soy sauce flavoured with lemon juice; a dash of teriyaki sauce; some ready-made mustard.

Protein sources

Many health experts in the UK, Japan and elsewhere agree that a healthy eating pattern for children and adults must include protein-rich foods such as fish, lean meat or poultry, and beans and lentils. In Japan, the most popular protein sources include fish, soya beans (eaten raw as edamame beans or as natto, a fermented version of soya beans), and tofu, which is a partly processed form of soya beans. Japanese families eat meat as well, but in smaller proportions than in the West. In the US, where I now live, for example, it seems that portion sizes for meat have got out of control, especially in many restaurants. In Japan, meat is enjoyed more as a garnish, a side dish or to add flavour rather than as the central feature of a big main course. The recipe section will show you some of these examples, and I hope you will be tempted to try them.

Healthy fats

Fat is not evil – not by any means. Fat helps food taste good. In recent years, unsaturated fats have been recognised as having distinct health benefits. According to many health experts, much or most of the fat that your family eats should come from unsaturated sources, which can improve blood cholesterol levels, ease inflammation, stabilise heart rhythms and provide other health benefits. There are two types of unsaturated fat sources: polyunsaturated and monounsaturated.

According to the Harvard School of Public Health, good sources of monounsaturated fats include olives, peanuts and rapeseed oils; avocados; nuts such as almonds, hazelnuts and pecan nuts; and seeds such as sesame and pumpkin seeds. Rapeseed oil and sesame seeds are particular favourites in Japan (more on this in the ingredients and recipe sections). Good sources of polyunsaturated fats are sunflower, corn, soybean and flaxseed oils, walnuts, flaxseeds, fish and rapeseed oil, which is a good source of both monounsaturated fat and polyunsaturated fat.

I have incorporated a number of traditionally non-Japanese ingredients containing healthy fats into my home-cooking.

Japanese-style rice: the belly-filling powerhouse

Japanese dietary patterns are based on much more rice than Western patterns: roughly ten times more than in the US and UK. Rice is the bedrock of many Asian diets, including Japan, where it is often served in its own little bowl, usually as a side dish, often even at breakfast.

Japanese-style short-grain rice, either brown or white, has a different taste from what you might be used to. You might find it quite delightful because it's moister, a bit sweeter and slightly stickier (but not gummy) than long-grain varieties. Its subtle flavour is a perfect companion for any of the dishes you serve. It has a naturally wonderful flavour and texture. It fills you up, gives you energy and leaves less room for less healthy foods such as biscuits and pastries.

Brown rice, which was Japan's original power food, is a great whole-grain, high-fibre choice and has a hearty and nutty flavour.

Why is rice, especially brown rice, so healthy?

I love brown rice, not only for its flavour, but also because it has much more fibre and nutrients than white rice. I enjoy short-grain white rice as well, because it tastes exquisitely delicious and was a pillar of the diet I grew up with, and I know it helps me fill up as part of my healthy meals, leaving almost no room to crave so-called junk foods. That's the part I like the most.

A note for parents of under-fives

You do have to be mindful of giving high-fibre foods to children under five. The NHS advice for children in this age group is to have a diet that is higher in fat and lower in fibre, with a good variety of fruit and veg. According to the NHS Choices website, 'Foods that contain a lot of fibre (such as wholemeal bread and pasta, brown rice and bran-based breakfast cereals) can fill up small tummies, leaving little room for other foods. This means that your child can get full before they've taken in the calories they need. Bran also prevents important minerals from being absorbed from the diet. It's good for your child to try different varieties of starchy foods, but don't give only wholegrain foods before your child is five years old.'

For more whole grains, replace refined cereal foods with whole-grain versions. Look for the word 'whole' before the name of the cereal, such as whole oats and whole-wheat pasta. In the absence of scientific/expert consensus recommendations on precise portion sizes, this should be left to parents and children to decide in a relaxed, natural fashion – always bearing in mind that grains are best regarded as a side dish.

Whole grains

Health experts advise us that grains are a healthy necessity in our diet, and that it's important to eat at least half our grains as whole grains. But what *is* a whole grain? And why does it matter?

Whole grains include grains such as wheat, corn, rice, oats, barley, quinoa, sorghum, spelt and rye eaten in their *whole* form (more on that later) – even popcorn is a whole grain! They are a good source of disease-fighting nutrients, phytochemicals and antioxidants, including B vitamins, vitamin E, magnesium, iron and fibre.

A whole grain contains all the essential parts and naturally occurring nutrients of the entire grain seed, in their original proportions if it has been processed (e.g., cracked, crushed, rolled, extruded and/or cooked). One hundred per cent of the original kernel – all of the bran, germ and endosperm – must be present to qualify as a whole grain. Each element of the grain contains nutrients.

The health benefits of whole grains

The medical evidence is clear that a diet rich in whole grains can reduce the risk of heart disease, stroke, cancer, diabetes and obesity. Few foods can offer such diverse benefits. People who eat whole grains regularly have a lower risk of obesity, as measured by their body mass index (BMI) and waist-to-hip ratios. They also have lower cholesterol levels.

Eating whole grains instead of refined grains lowers the risk of many chronic diseases. While the benefits are most pronounced for those consuming at least three servings daily, some studies show reduced risks from as little as one serving daily. The message: every whole grain in your diet helps!

The benefits of whole grains most documented by studies include better weight maintenance and reducing the risks of stroke, type-2 diabetes, heart disease and certain forms of cancer. Other benefits suggested by recent studies include: reduced risk of asthma, healthier carotid arteries, reduction of inflammatory disease risk, lower risk of colorectal cancer, healthier blood pressure levels and less gum disease and tooth loss.

Increasing the consumption of whole grains should be done progressively, however, to let the body adapt to a higher fibre content, and not before the age of five years, as explained on page 39.

Shopping for whole-grain foods

When buying whole grains, whether loose or in other foods, look out for the word 'whole' as in 'wholemeal', 'whole grain' or '100 per cent wholemeal/or whole-wheat' on the packaging. Remember to look for choices with minimal added sugars – a whole oat flapjack that's smothered in syrup is still a sugary treat.

The following are useful whole-grain choices: porridge made with oats or oatmeal, whole-grain cereals, such as muesli, that are sugar-free, rye bread (pumpernickel), wholemeal, Granary, wheatgerm or mixed-grain breads, whole-wheat crackers, rye crackers and crispbreads, whole-grain rice cakes and oatcakes. When choosing flours, look for wholemeal flour, wheatgerm, buckwheat flour, unrefined rye and barley flour, oatmeal and oat flour. To serve with meals, look for brown rice, whole-wheat pasta, pot and pearl barley, bulgur wheat and quinoa.

The bottom line

As explained at the beginning of the chapter, tweak the family diet – enjoy a family food pattern that is higher in nutrients, includes more plant-based foods like fruit and vegetables and whole grains, as well as fish, and have less processed food and added sugars and salt. This kind of diet is generally agreed by dieticians and experts on family health as being an excellent model to aim for.

Celebrate Food Joy and Flexible Restraint

Practise flexible restraint, not severe food
restriction or food demonisation.

———————

Mummy?
Yes, child?
Mummy smells nice. It's the smell of the omelette you
were just cooking, isn't it?

Japanese nursery song

The Japan I grew up in was, and still is, a land in love with healthy and delicious food. The food markets were, as they are today, overflowing with fresh, sinfully succulent produce and choice cuts of beef and fish, mothers and housewives exchanged tips on finding the freshest, most beautiful produce, and at night the side streets of our Tokyo residential district were redolent with the aromas of home-cooked miso soup with tofu chunks, simmered carrots, gobo burdock, daikon radish and shiitake mushrooms in dashi cooking broth, grilled mackerel fillets and nutty soba noodles.

Japan has long been joyfully obsessed with fresh, healthy food, and children are often taught from birth both by their parents as well as their schools to understand how food is grown, prepared and ritually eaten. My own mother, Chizuko, is a prime example of a generation of so-called kitchen-goddess mothers who came of age in Japan in the rapidly industrialising post-war years of the 1950s and 1960s. At the time, both Asian and Western food, as well as modern appliances, became abundant, but the country still stayed closely connected to a culture of very healthy eating patterns.

My mother encouraged our family to enjoy a wonderfully healthy eating pattern centred on generous helpings of veggies from the land, sea and mountains, and fresh fruit, fish and rice. She also encouraged us to enjoy occasional treats, snacks and sugar – but in the proper amounts and frequencies, which are much smaller and less frequent than in the West.

In other words, she led us to follow a lifelong pattern of food joy when it came to healthy food, and flexible restraint when it came to less healthy food – not severe food restriction or food demonisation. Also, in our house, as in many Japanese homes, there was much less worktop and cupboard space to store large amounts of less-healthy foods and snacks compared to many Western homes, and therefore much less of a practice of hiding such items far out of reach of children, a tactic that probably backfires by focusing children's attention and desire for the foods. The lesson might be: just don't bring the less-healthy stuff home! As leading child-feeding researcher Dr Leann Birch put it, 'Take the kid out for ice cream once or twice a week, but don't keep it in the house.'

Mealtime problems – they occur in Japan, too

Things are not perfect in the kingdom of healthy longevity. At the Kaji Sakura Nursery School in Hokkaido, a group of Japanese mothers is having a group nutrition therapy session with the school nutritionist.

The mothers are worried.

They're having trouble helping their children become healthy eaters. Even though they live in the nation that is the world capital of healthy longevity, and the food habits of Japanese children are very good overall, these women have learned that there are still plenty of picky eaters, vegetable-refusers and food-throwers among them.

'My child doesn't eat at all!' says one mother.

'My child eats so slowly compared to other children,' despairs another.

'Really? Mine, too! As soon as my child starts eating, she gets bored and escapes from the baby chair.'

'Mine, too! Plus, my child spills food, terribly. When I look at the floor after a meal, I'm horrified.'

'My child eats anything. That's great, but he doesn't stop. How about a child who keeps eating?'

The school nutritionist, Tomomi Takahashi, listens quietly as the mothers pour out a barrage of emotions. She can relate to what's being said; she's a mother herself. She's heard many of these concerns before, and felt some of them herself with her own children.

When everyone has vented their emotions and anecdotes, all eyes turn to Ms Takahashi. Gently, she begins to reveal the tips of a Japanese mother and nutrition professional who has worked with the food habits of hundreds of school children over the years, as well as her own. She says, 'It's important to think about your child's eating habits in the long term. A child's habits don't change overnight. A child's interests and taste for foods change. Dislikes can become likes when a meal environment or the way food is served changes.

'If a child has little appetite, or takes a long time to eat, it's a natural behaviour, it's just who the child naturally is.'

The emotions are flowing freely, interspersed with moments of polite laughter when the mums realise they're facing many of the same child-feeding problems.

'Please understand your child's feelings. Don't talk down to him or her. Only the child knows why they like or dislike a food. Remember your own childhood? Certainly you had foods you didn't like. Perhaps, you still have some.'

At this, I smiled in recognition. While I remember being a relatively good eater as a child, every day in the late afternoon, I would ask, 'What's for dinner, Mama? I'm getting hungry.' Often, her answer was 'fish', and I would try to persuade her to serve something else. It wasn't that I disliked the flavours or textures of fish, I found the process of separating flesh from bones, especially fine ones, a tedious nuisance. In Japan, fish is often cooked and served whole, including the bones, and for me, fish for dinner was a bummer. Then, one day in my early teens, with no warning, I snapped out of this rejective mode and suddenly I liked fish!

Ms Takahashi continues, 'Children keenly sense the feelings and thoughts of parents and people around them. Just because a child doesn't eat something, don't get frustrated and try forcing him to eat. That will have a completely negative effect. If you force a child to eat something, they may avoid it later on. Even if a child could eat something just because a parent or a teacher talked him into it on one occasion, he won't feel like eating it next time.'

Mistakes we make with children's eating

As I absorbed Ms Takahashi's words, I was embarrassed to realise that I was sometimes guilty of making some of these same mistakes myself with my own young child, of applying pressure and stress to his eating experience.

Parents sometimes have the urge to say things like, 'Eat your greens or there's no TV', 'Have just another bite of carrots and then you can have dessert', 'No more carbs – carbs make you fat', or this, always at a children's party: 'The kids are eating too much sugar – that's what's making them so wild and jumpy!'

Then I remembered two of the strangest things I heard of a parent telling a child. The first case was in an American supermarket, when a slightly overweight girl of about 12 stopped in front of the baked goods section and told her mother she wanted a cupcake. The mother leaned down and declared, 'That does it, young lady – you're going on a *diet!*'

Another time, in a playground not far from our home in

Manhattan, a girl asked her father if they could get an ice cream from an ice cream truck parked right outside the playground. The father replied with a quiet, thoughtful litany: 'No, dear, you know we can't. The ice cream would spike your blood sugar, and then you'd get overweight, and then you'd get obese, and then you'd get diabetes, and then we'd have to take you to the doctor, then we'd have to put you in a hospital.' The mother, standing nearby, nodded firmly in support. All this from an ice cream! The parents' hearts were probably in the right place, but they appeared to be doing the exact opposite of what the experts recommend to promote healthy eating habits in children.

As one New York mother, Harriet Brown, wrote in the *New York Times* on 30 May 2006: 'Early in my children's lives, I was a no-sugar, no-fat mom, the legacy of my own childhood with a constantly dieting mother. I thought I was doing the right thing, until a friend told me that every time my children stayed at her house, the first thing they did was ask for ice cream. With sprinkles. And chocolate chips. And gummy worms. By rigidly restricting their sugar intake, I had made it a highly sought-out pleasure – the last thing I'd intended.'

Relax and make mealtimes enjoyable times

Back at the Kaji Sakura Nursery School in Hokkaido, nutritionist Ms Takahashi has some great advice for all parents. 'Relax,' she said. 'You don't need to try so hard. Have a relaxed attitude and mind, so your child can relax and be comfortable eating. Show your child that you enjoy eating, and the food tastes wonderful.

'There is nothing sadder than eating a meal alone. Even when you're busy, please set a specific meal time so you can sit down and eat with your child at least once a day.' She continues, 'Cook your meals with love, and it will resonate in the child's heart. Feel the joy of eating together with your child.'

Ms Takahashi may not necessarily know it, but the bits of wisdom she shared have been validated by some of the world's leading experts. Her tips, in fact, are among the world's most effective, research-based, cutting-edge advice on the subject of children's food habits, and getting your child to enjoy a healthy eating pattern.

In Japan, as in many other cultures, food is seen as a celebration of life, family, joy, love and health. What is interesting about Japan, in my experience, is that, even with the experiences of the mothers at the Kaji Sakura Nursery School, and even with a real problem of young women in Japan who suffer from excessive thinness, the overall traditional Japanese food culture, when compared with that in the urbanised West, is closer to the traditional Mediterranean food culture: more relaxed, less stressful, more focused on the ritualised joy of eating delicious, healthy food and much less focused on the 'shame' of eating 'bad foods' and 'forbidden foods'. In Japan, however, sugar, for example, is usually not seen as much as an enemy but something to be enjoyed – just not in the amounts consumed in the West.

The emerging research on child-feeding psychology strongly supports the thinking of the Japanese school nutritionist Ms Takahashi, and the practices of many Japanese parents and smart parents around the world. Japan is far from perfect by any means, but I've noticed that many Japanese children are taught to practise joy and flexible restraint when it comes to food, not severe food restriction or food demonisation, and they are supported by parents who communicate food and lifestyle wisdom in an authori*tative* rather than authori*tarian* style.

Breaking news: startling new research on children and healthy eating

In a series of experiments, studies and discoveries that have unfolded over the past two decades at institutions in the UK, the US and elsewhere, researchers have come to some stark, surprising and sometimes sharply counterintuitive observations. In a nutshell, the research suggests that parents should 'lighten up' about their children's eating habits, cut out food stress and pressure, and consider doing much the opposite of what many parents do.

When my husband and I first learned of this research, we were stunned. Somehow, despite the fact that I was raised in a super-healthy family food culture, and despite multiple paediatrician check-up visits, piles of parenting books and magazines, and countless hours of playground talk with other parents, we had not clearly heard many of these messages before.

In a December 2011 paper in the journal *Appetite* ('Development of healthy eating habits early in life: Review of recent evidence and selected guidelines'), researchers analysed the available research on encouraging healthy eating habits from the beginning of complementary feeding until the age of three years. They found that the 'authoritative-democratic' style, or providing overall rules, and setting a relaxed, confident example and a positive context, is associated with the development of the healthiest feeding habits. They also found that there is a 'relative consensus' in the research that 'too much parental control (i.e. pressuring and restricting) has negative consequences', but they were quick to point out that 'since most studies on this aspect were carried out with white American middle to higher SES [socioeconomic status] girls, whether such findings can be generalized to other socio-economic classes, to other ethnicities or to boys is questionable'.

William and I had to find out more. Maybe we could learn something that could help our own family, so we searched out the best expert advice we could find, and we talked to some of the experts around the world who are doing the best research in the field of healthy eating for children. While common patterns are emerging in the research, a major caveat is that it is in its relatively early stages, and much more research needs to be done, especially with children of different cultures, ethnicities and income groups. But here's what the emerging research suggests:

- Some parents are excessively pressuring their children to eat healthy foods, and over-restricting or demonising certain foods with blanket oversimplifications like 'sugar is bad for you!' or 'carbs make you fat!'.

- Telling a child to 'clean their plate' can lead the child to dislike the foods he or she is being pressured to eat, whereas too-strict control of the child's diet can lead to overeating. Children who had been told to clean their plates were much less responsive to food cues than children who had been taught to focus on internal cues, such as feeling hungry or full. Most infants and young children seem to have the capacity to self-regulate their own calorie intake.

- Pressure on a child to eat can create a dislike for certain foods on the one hand and can disrupt his or her ability to regulate food intake on the other. Food over-restriction can encourage children to eat when they aren't hungry.

As child-feeding specialist Dr Lucy Cooke puts it, 'Some restriction is necessary – it's the total ban on certain foods that backfires.' Highly controlling practices, it seems, may undermine a child's ability to develop and exercise self-control over his or her own eating:

- Overtly and very strictly limiting a child's intake of a certain food is more likely to cause the child to want the item that much more. Restricting access to a food that's in the house focuses children's attention on the restricted food, while increasing their desire to obtain and consume it.

- Paradoxically, the process goes awry when well-intentioned parents start imposing control over when and how much their children eat, like focusing on what's left on their plates rather than letting the child decide when he's had enough.

- Parents should be responsible for selecting the foods for children to eat, but it should be up to the child to decide how much. Adults should trust their children's ability to regulate their own food intakes.

- Parents should learn to trust kids when they say they're hungry or full. Pressure to eat by over-aggressively promoting healthy food, usually fruit and vegetables, restriction by limiting access to sweets and fatty snacks kept in the house, and the use of food as a reward, are associated with negative outcomes; restriction is strongly correlated with children's 'disinhibited' eating behaviours. Restriction is also directly associated with higher children's body mass index (BMI).

- Food restriction by mothers can promote overeating, especially in daughters. In one study, girls who were already overweight at five years of age and who received higher levels of restriction also had the highest tendency to eat when they weren't hungry.

- Authoritarian feeding practices usually backfire. As the authors of a December 2011 paper in the medical journal *Pediatric Clinics of North America* ('Etiologies of obesity in children: Nature and nurture') found, 'Authoritarian parenting styles, characterized by restriction, pressures to eat certain foods, and over-monitoring, are most consistently linked to pediatric weight gain.'

The media don't help either. For years, the messages we all got as parents and as consumers, often from misreported science, or oversimplified government guidelines, seemed to be 'fat and carbs make you fat' and 'sugar is poison'. The actual science, however, is pointing toward a more nuanced, and healthy, conclusion – 'good (unsaturated) fats and good (unrefined, complex) carbs (like whole grains) and naturally-occurring sugars (like those in fruit) are important parts of a healthy eating pattern for children and adults'.

What all this research points to is something that many parents in Japan and the UK have known all along – that a positive, authoritative approach is best, rather than a punitive, authoritarian approach. As dietician Connie Evers has put it, 'The parent's role is to offer a variety of healthful foods, oversee the planning and assembly of meals, and set the schedule for meals and snacks. The child's responsibility is to decide what, how much, and even whether to eat.'

Be relaxed about less-healthy food

When it comes to snacks at home, you could say Japan has been a lucky victim of architecture: many Japanese kitchens have little extra storage space, and nowhere to put large quantities of crisps and biscuits. Japanese children enjoy snacks, but in smaller quantities and frequencies than many children in the West.

The tip, for parents, may be simple. Rather than bring the big bags of biscuits and crisps home and hide them out of reach only to endure children pleading for them, just don't keep them in the house! Instead, why not enjoy small portions of sweets or chocolate with your children once or twice a week or a few times a month, perhaps away from home. And as *New York Times* reporter Tara Parker-Pope has suggested, don't buy fizzy drinks, sweets and crisps and then put them on a high shelf in the cupboard. Instead, stock up with healthy foods, and then you can allow your children access and a reasonable amount of control over what they eat. For a snack, give them the choice of an apple or orange or vegetables with different dips.

Many experts suggest that relaxed, moderate restraint toward less-healthy food, rather than rigid, frequent restriction – an idea you could call 'flexible restraint' – can be a rewarding path towards healthy eating in children. Leading Australian dietician Rosemary Stanton agrees, 'No food should be demonized. Everything is OK occasionally. However, note that "occasionally" is an inappropriate term for a three year old who will always think "occasionally" is "now".' Dr David L. Katz, MD, of the Yale University School of Medicine told me 'flexible restraint is a natural result of habituating to wholesome foods. All of the effort involved in eating well tends to go away when you learn to love foods that love you back in the first place.' In New Delhi, leading obesity and diabetes experts Prof. Anoop Misra and Dr Seema Gulati told us, 'Being very strict is only going to increase the craving for junk food. Flexible restraint works better as it teaches children self-discipline, which helps them throughout their lives.' And as Penn State nutritionist Jennifer Orlet Fisher once put it,

'There's nothing wrong with watching what children eat and making sure they eat well. But if you're looking to promote good dietary habits, moderation and judicious choices may be better than strict rules.'

Aim to emphasise enjoyment

Back at the Kaji Sakura Nursery School in Hokkaido, nutritionist Ms Takahashi reveals to her fellow Japanese mothers the idea that she considers to be the most critical insight she has yet discovered on the subject of helping to nurture a healthy child: 'The important thing is that your child enjoys eating and she or he looks forward to a meal time. To enjoy a meal and to feed himself with his own initiative is the number-one secret for the child's healthy growth.'*

The lesson: practise flexible restraint, not severe food restriction or food demonisation.

* Source for Kaji Sukura Nursery School story: Cabinet Office, Government of Japan, 'Shokuiku Textbook for Parents and Children' http://www8.cao.go.jp/syokuiku/data/textbook/index.html (Japanese)

Inspire Your Child to Enjoy New Foods

Gently encourage your children to try to enjoy a wide variety of different healthy foods, including many different fruits and vegetables.

———————

Children grow up watching their parents' backs.
Japanese saying

You are at the family dinner table. You've prepared a beautiful bowl of steamed spinach. You want your child to get in the habit of eating healthy food, and you've decided that today is the day, and the time is now. 'Try it,' you tell your child, 'it's delicious. It's good for you!' Your child takes a look, and scrunches up her face. 'Come on,' you beseech her, 'it's really delicious!'

'No!' Not a chance. Her lips are locked shut and her arms are folded. She shakes her head. She may be responding to a distant, genetically programmed biological human instinct that associates bitter tastes to potential toxins. Or she may be responding in solidarity with her schoolmates, who had the same reaction to a lunch-tray full of greens earlier that day. No matter. This is simply not going to happen. The spinach will not be eaten.

It is a scene repeated countless times a day, all around the world, even in Japan. And it is an unfortunate reality: foods that kids like the most are usually the least nutritious. Surveys of children across cultures, including France, Germany and America, have revealed common favourites: French fries, chocolate, pizza, cake and ice cream; and a common least favourite: vegetables. Many children seem to suffer from what experts call 'neophobia', or the reluctance to taste unfamiliar foods, which often arises around the age of two and gradually declines after the preschool years.

Paving the way to healthy eating

What then, does work? How can we actually persuade our children to eat in the healthiest way possible? How can you persuade a child to eat healthy foods and adopt a healthy eating pattern that's more similar to the Japanese national eating pattern, with fewer empty calories and more good stuff like fish and vegetable produce? How can you effect positive changes to your child's lifestyle?

At first, it may seem totally impossible. Let's face it, as parents, we live in the real world, where children seem genetically engineered to dislike vegetables and prefer pizza, biscuits and tons of sugar; where children are bombarded with fast-food ads, unhealthy choices and bad role models everywhere; where daily exercise seems impossible, and where many families can barely find the time to get enough sleep and get out the door on time in the morning, much less find any time for home cooking.

In Japan, it is easier to expose children to an overall healthier eating pattern, since it is more the national norm than in many other developed nations, in homes, in schools and in eating out. But in many Western and Westernising food cultures, the cultural and social biases that children may feel against healthier eating patterns may seem stronger, so many parents may need to try harder. In the UK and the US, for example, many parents have lost the time or the impulse to cook at home, and processed and prepared foods, that are often less healthy, have taken over the family table.

There is, however, some great news.

Prolong your child's life with a new food

In food research laboratories at the University of Pennsylvania and University College London, teams of researchers are working out how, in effect, to help children enjoy an eating pattern that is more like the Japanese pattern or any other healthy, more traditional pattern, with more vegetable products, more fish and more sensible amounts of calories consumed.

The scientists are unlocking the keys to an exquisitely complex and incredibly difficult question: how can we get our children to fall in love with a wide variety of healthy foods? The solution is incredibly important, because research has found that the number of healthy foods tried by a child between the ages of two and eight has a direct impact on the child's future health. As the authors of an August 2007 paper ('The importance of exposure for healthy eating in childhood') in the *Journal of Human Nutrition and Diet* put it, 'research suggests that the earlier and broader that experience, the healthier the child's diet'.

The scientists are coming to a series of often surprising conclusions, which many Japanese children already know and experience in their daily lives, because Japanese parents are able to adopt a healthier overall family eating pattern from the birth of their children. This research is largely still new, and much more work needs to be done, but here is what it is suggesting:

- Children's food likes and dislikes change over time, and parents can gently steer them towards healthier patterns, by exposing them to a wide variety of choices and by setting an example.

- The earlier and wider a child's experience with sampling new healthy foods, the healthier their diet will become through childhood. Repeated opportunities for a child to sample new foods leads to their trying more, eating more and liking more. Most parents of older children know this already, and many mothers will have discovered this already for themselves. This insight can inspire you to continue to tempt your children with new tastes through their childhood, because their taste can mature, expand and change constantly as they grow up – right into adulthood.

As Dr Silvia Scaglioni of the University of Milan and her colleagues wrote in a 2011 paper ('Determinants of children's eating behavior', *American Journal of Clinical Nutrition*, December 2011), parents can reduce, or even reverse, their child's dislike for a food by providing adequate food and portion sizes at mealtimes and promoting social interaction and themselves as role models for eating behaviours. They added, 'research suggests that the earlier and broader experiences with food are, the healthier is the child's diet'. In one study, food neophobia, or fear of the new, early in life was related to the number of foods disliked or never tried by the age of eight.

If a parent 'gives up' on exposing their child to unfamiliar foods, they may reinforce the child's aversion to trying foods. For a food to become accepted it should be offered a number of times, and ideally, early in life. Two- to six-year-old children had a higher frequency of consumption of vegetables and fruit when they were exposed to them early. Giving a new food a familiar flavour, like a dip, ketchup or curry, can increase a child's interest in trying it. And this practice can be encouraged through childhood, to steer a child towards a lifetime of enjoying new foods. As my grandmother Tsune often said, echoing a bit of Japanese folk wisdom, 'a new food prolongs one's life'.

When is the right time to start?

The start of weaning appears to be an ideal time to try to introduce new foods, especially vegetables. Between five and seven months, many early reactions to new foods are positive and even sour or bitter-tasting foods are accepted. Food neophobia appears around the age of two and is associated with lower dietary variety and quality.

Infants may need only one exposure to a new food to sharply

increase their eating and liking it; and children over two years old might need significantly more – up to 20 exposures in one study of 7–9 and 10–12-year-olds. But many parents may be giving up much too early. As the European Network for Public Health Nutrition explained in 2006:

> It is important that children, for whom all complementary foods are initially unfamiliar, have repeated exposure to new foods during the early complementary feeding period in order to establish a healthy food acceptance pattern. It has been suggested that a minimum of 8–10 exposures are needed, with clear increases in food acceptance appearing after 12–15 exposures.

What are the lessons? To translate the research into common-sense 'mum's advice':

- Don't give up! Keep offering your child samples of new foods in a no-pressure way.

- Let them see you enjoying new and healthy foods.

- Remember that your child's tastes change, and a food they hate today could be a food they try and love tomorrow.

- To help your child be adventurous you can make mixtures of vegetables, such as a ratatouille (or try one of the Japanese-style veggie recipes at the end of this book), or serve vegetables in soups, which can make them palatable and more exciting than simply served alone.

Children eat what the family eats

Preparing a separate 'kids meal' of special foods and dishes for children who are developmentally ready to eat family foods is usually a bad idea, as it unintentionally delays and discourages children from joining the natural rhythm of family meals. Repeatedly and gently exposing a child to new foods and setting a good example are more effective than applying coercion or pressure. For families who follow healthy 'traditional' styles of Japanese, Asian, Mediterranean, UK or other European eating patterns, 'kid's menus' and 'kid's foods' are a non-starter – children eat what the family eats, as soon as they are developmentally ready. And remember to keep trying, and not give up too early.

In a paper in the Spring 2007 issue of the *Journal of Law, Medicine and Ethics* ('Parental influence on eating behaviour: Conception to adolescence'), researchers, Jennifer S. Savage, Jennifer Orlet Fisher and Leann L. Birch, concluded, 'New foods may need to be offered to preschool-aged children 10 to 16 times before acceptance occurs. At the same time, simply offering new foods will not necessarily produce liking; having children taste new foods is a necessary part of the process. Awareness of this normal course of food acceptance is important because approximately one-quarter of parents with infants and toddlers prematurely drew conclusions about their child's preference for foods after [only] two or fewer exposures.'

How to encourage tasting and sampling

Let's go back to your dinner table, and your child's dish of uneaten spinach.

If one of the most important keys to guiding your child to a healthy eating pattern is getting her to sample a wide variety of new foods, you are still faced with a huge challenge – how do you do it? If you've offered a sample to them many times and they still decide not to try it, how do you get the new food in their mouth so that they will at least taste it? Frankly stated, there is more than one expert opinion on this. For widely respected dietician and psychotherapist Ellyn Satter, for example, it's all about a division of responsibility. The parent's responsibility is to choose and prepare the foods, and the child's responsibility is to decide how much and which to eat of the choices given. Eventually, Satter believes, they will come to like the foods you like, as long as pressure, coercion and parental attempts at control are removed from the process.

Many mothers in Japan, the UK and elsewhere have also dis-covered that a child may not like a plainly cooked veg on its own, but they might eat it in some other form or as part of a meal – a veggie-rich tomato sauce, a veggie burger, a fruit-and-veggie packed smoothie, or a baked sweet potato, cooked like chips or French fries as a side dish or snack. Many Japanese mums put chopped fish, meat and a wide variety of vegetables into steamed short-grain rice for their children to enjoy.

There is also a fascinating new approach to helping your child sample new foods in a no-pressure environment, an approach pioneered by Dr Lucy Cooke of University College London and her colleagues. Dr Cooke, who has been studying children's feed-ing habits for over 20 years, calls the approach Tiny Tastes, and you can think of it as giving 'smart rewards' to your children for sampling new foods. Her programme involves the judicious use of something kids love: stickers.

When I first heard of Dr Cooke's idea to use stickers as a gentle, low-key, fun, smart reward to help children sample healthy new foods, I smiled. I remembered my own childhood in Japan, where I, and millions of other Japanese children, were given stickers as rewards in a nationwide campaign to encourage a radio-delivered exercise programme every day of the summer holidays. The programme, called *rajio taiso*, is still widely used in Japan today.

In thinking of a way to help children sample new fruits and vegetables, Dr Cooke reviewed the research on using rewards. She knew that the idea of using rewards with children was somewhat controversial in the research community, because if a reward is too significant it can undermine a child's intrinsic motivation. As she puts it, 'the reward should help the child do something, but they shouldn't be doing it just to get the reward'. The ingenious solution was to use stickers and to reward the children not for liking the food but for tasting the food and giving their opinion of it. The power of deciding whether or not to like the food is left entirely up to the child and the reward is given just for tasting a new fruit or vegetable. Even if the child spits it out, they still get a sticker. Cooke and her colleagues realised that 'where intake is the outcome, the effects of rewards tend to be positive' but 'where liking is the outcome, results are mixed'. Hence, the emphasis on trying, but not necessarily liking.

In a study that lasted over three months with three- to six-year-olds in London nursery schools, the Tiny Tastes programme produced significant, sustained increases in children's liking of various new vegetables, including carrot, cucumber, white cabbage, red pepper, celery and sugar snap peas. The results were published in the January 2012 issue of the *American Journal of Clinical Nutrition*, with an explanation of how the programme worked:

> Different vegetables can be offered over time, but parents are encouraged to focus on one at a time for each 14-day period. To begin, the parent selects a moderately disliked or unfamiliar vegetable for the child to try. At a set time each day (e.g., snack time or just before a meal), the parent presents the vegetable (whole, if possible) to the child, talks about where the vegetable comes from or how it grows, and prepares it in front of the child. The parent then asks the child to taste a small piece of the vegetable, without any seasonings, dips, or dressings. Each time the child tastes the vegetable, the parent rewards the child with tangible non-food items (checkmark on a chart and a sticker) as well as verbal praise. This process is repeated with the same vegetable for 14 days.

Parents were asked to be neutral if a child refused to taste a vegetable or disliked it. To the child, it seems like a fun tasting game with the promise of earning a sticker.

Dr Cooke and her colleagues reported that most of the parents in the study had positive comments, like, 'The tide has turned!', 'She ate the whole piece and said "I like celery"', 'She got her sticker. Then she asked for another piece and said she loved it. Wow!' Another parent said, 'It's the best piece of advice I've been given.' The researchers concluded, 'The "Tiny Tastes" program may provide a novel and practical strategy to help parents achieve a healthier diet for their children.'

I've recently tried this Japanese-style idea with my own son to help him sample new foods, and it worked very well. In practice, it seemed to be a gentle, effective approach. Renowned children's food researcher Dr Leann Birch loves the approach. She told us, 'I think this is a great idea; one of the reasons kids refuse to taste new foods is that they are afraid they will "taste bad". Finding non-coercive ways to help children learn to take a taste, try new things, and learn that they don't taste bad is a step in the right direction.'

Dr Cooke believes that the Tiny Tastes method 'takes the anxiety away' from a dinner table process that can get very chaotic and anxiety producing. 'With this approach, mums feel they know exactly what they're doing, the child knows exactly what they're doing. There's no need to get upset. If it doesn't work today, the mum and the child know you can just try again tomorrow. Don't worry if the child spits it out, it's fine, as long as he's managed to taste it.' She believes the programme, which you can find out more about at www.weightconcern.org.uk/tinytastes, can work for most children from about the age of three upwards.

Dr Cooke adds, 'I think Tiny Tastes should work for any age provided that they still like stickers. In general though, repeated tasting works to increase liking in any age group for any food type with or without a sticker (or any other kind of) reward. For example, adults who take sugar in their coffee may find the taste of coffee without sugar unpleasant, but if they persevere and drink it without sugar for 10–15 days, they will come to prefer it that way. It's magic!'

20 Japanese mum's tips ...

... for helping children to fall in love with healthy eating.

Based on my interviews with scores of Japanese mums, and on the opinions of a number of global experts on child feeding, here are some mum-and-dad-tested tips for helping your child enjoy healthy food:

1   Don't necessarily call it 'healthy food'. There is some intriguing new research suggesting that labelling food as 'healthy' or 'power-food' can focus a child's opposition to it. Instead, make nutrient-rich, less-processed foods and meals rich in vegetables, fruit and whole grains be the normal routine in your home.

2   Serve vegetable soups and stir-fries as a regular option at the dinner table – they are a great way to boost the family veg intake, and children often love them.

3   Don't demonise high-calorie/nutrient-poor snacks such as biscuits, crisps, ice cream, sweets, cakes and corn chips – just keep them mostly out of the house and let your child enjoy them occasionally in small portions, ideally away from home. In the words of a Japanese saying, 'There is no evil in food one likes to eat.'

4   Make veg and fruit your family's default snack – try apple slices, mandarin/orange segments, banana pennies, carrot sticks, celery sticks, avocado slices, baked sweet potato 'chips'.

5   Make fruit the default dessert in your house for yourself and your children.

6   Stock your kitchen with a wide variety of fresh, frozen and canned fruit and veg.

7   Put whole or blended veggies into pasta and pizza sauces and tacos; shred courgettes or carrots into spaghetti Bolognese, casseroles, quick breads and muffins; chop veggies into lasagne; use puréed, cooked vegetables, such as potatoes, to thicken gravies, stews and soups. Veggies add texture, nutrients and a great flavour to all kinds of dishes and meals. It's not a case of hiding vegetables in a child's meals, but more about offering them meals with more flavour and more ingredients.

8   Many vegetables taste great with a dip or dressing. Try offering your child pieces of raw or lightly steamed broccoli, baby carrots, sugar snap peas, celery sticks, red and green peppers, or cauliflower with a dip such as a modest portion of olive oil, hummus, yoghurt with no added sugar, or a salad dressing. Children love to eat foods with their fingers, and they love to dip.

9   Decorate plates or serving dishes with fun-shaped vegetable slices or fingers.

10 Take your child to markets to see the wide range of vegetables there are, and ask your child to pick out a few items to take home.

11 Involve your child in preparing, washing and serving food. You can buy fun aprons for them to wear.

12 If you have a garden, involve your child in growing some vegetables. If you don't have a garden, try growing herbs in pots on the windowsill or grow cress in eggshells or on a pad of cotton wool – they can even create a garden in a shallow plastic container using pebbles or stones.

13 When you're in the supermarket, ask your child to pick out a new food for the whole family to try.

14 Offer your child healthy foods as a part of a normal, relaxed routine.

15 Keep mealtimes a pleasant experience. Remember that children's tastes change, and the foods they hate one day can become favourites the next.

16 Don't pressure your child to eat certain foods and don't let mealtimes become a 'battle' because this will make mealtimes into an emotional drama. Be aware that there will always be foods that they're not going to eat.

17 Do not use food as a reward for good behaviour.

18 Don't demand that your child cleans his or her plate.

19 Have set meal times, for stability and regularity. It makes sense to have these rituals in family life.

20 Try cooking methods that can bring out veggie flavours in a way that children can enjoy, such as roasting. Also try raw veggies.

Rebalance the Family Plate – With Japanese-style Portions

Serve food on modest-sized plates –
and don't skimp on the fruit and veggies!

———————

For a small vessel, use a small sail.

Japanese saying

In 2013, the British Heart Foundation (BHF) released a report that found that the average serving sizes of ready meals had contributed to the obesity crisis and had grown 'out of control' over the previous 20 years: a chicken curry with rice was 53 per cent bigger; a shepherd's pie was almost double; spaghetti Bolognese was 25 per cent bigger; macaroni and cheese was 39 per cent bigger; and crumpets, bagels and garlic bread were 20 per cent to 30 per cent larger. BHF chief executive Simon Gillespie declared, 'We urgently need a government review of portion sizes in the UK.' Dr Susan Jebb, professor of diet and population health at University of Oxford, has observed, 'There is no getting away from the fact that we are eating bigger portions ... I think it does matter. If you offer people larger portions, they eat more. They not only eat more at meals but they do not necessarily feel any fuller, nor do they eat less later on.'

In the UK, the US and elsewhere, competition among food and restaurant companies has driven them to offer larger portions, and we're gradually losing control of what a portion size should look like. The problem is that there appears to be a direct connection between the amount of food that's placed in front of us and the amount we over-consume. 'Studies show that people tend to passively overeat by about 25 per cent,' explained Prof. James Hill, of the University of Colorado. 'In other words, three-quarters of the way through a big bowl of pasta, you may be perfectly satisfied. But if there's more in the bowl, you'll eat it.'

A simple, super-easy solution

If you were to visit a traditional Japanese family home for dinner tonight, many of the foods you saw on the table might appear different from what you have at home, but closer examination would reveal that most of the dishes are made of the same food ingredients you're accustomed to in your life. There would be a few important differences, however: you'd be offered an optional pair of chopsticks, and dishes, plates and bowls would be smaller than you're used to. A bowl of miso soup would be served together with the meal, and most foods would be presented in their own small dishes. You'd be encouraged to take a bite of one food, then another, then some rice, and to gradually take little bites of each food in a relaxed rotation. The meat portion would be smaller, the proportion of vegetables higher.

A Japanese food portion is typically served in a moderate size on its own individual small plate. In fact, there's really no main course as such, but a satisfying variety of tastes and textures in manageable sizes: rice in a rice bowl, miso soup in a soup bowl, simmered vegetables in a bowl or plate, sea vegetable salad with rice vinegar dressing in a little bowl, a fillet of fish on a plate. Dishes such as noodles with toppings in a delicious broth are served in bowls that are 10–20 per cent smaller than their Western counterparts.

The overall calorie load of the Japanese-style meal would be lower than the typical Western-style meal, but it would be just as filling and satisfying. And the pattern of foods consumed would be closer in many ways to meeting the nutritional recommendations of many global health authorities than the typical Western meal. In Japan, portion sizes for foods prepared at home and away from home have remained pretty constant over the past decades – that's just the way the food culture has developed.

In this way of presenting family foods, Japan has a possible lesson for your family and the rest of the world. To help boost your children's health (and your own) rebalance the family meal with Japanese-style plates and portions, and serve food on modest-sized plates in reasonable portion sizes – and don't skimp on the fruit and veggies!

A new way of looking at serving food

I suggest you consider giving your larger serving plates a break and serve your family meals instead on smaller Japan-style plates, like the side plates and bowls you may already have – plates about 10–15cm (4–6in) in diameter, and the bowls about 3–10cm, holding about 100–200ml. To put this into context, a family meal served 'Japanese-style' might consist of soup, a small bowl of brown rice, four small plates: stir-fried vegetables; baked sweet potato fries; a portion of canned Alaskan salmon (or meat or tofu); and fruit for dessert.

The simple but powerful idea of serving food to children on smaller plates has appealed to Duncan Selbie, the chief executive of Public Health England, who in the 2 October 2014 *Newcastle Journal* told of meeting a mother who had been raised on the idea that one should always clear ones plate. 'The child [her son] was overweight at school, and it was a definite problem', reported Selbie, but the simple 'prescription' was to eat from smaller plates. Health experts in the north-east have supported the strategy of using smaller plates to fight rising obesity levels.

'We are seeing younger and younger children who are already seriously overweight,' reported dietician Hannah Mayer.

This can be before they have even started school. In the work we do with families in Gateshead we look at all ages of children and try to help the whole family make the changes they need to. Eating smaller portions of food is a really important message. A four-year-old does not need as much to eat as their 14-year-old brother. Small changes can make a big difference.

Dr Anne Dale, paediatrician at Gateshead Health NHS Foundation Trust, said:

> It is easy to eat unhealthy food, and most of us will tend to eat more than we need – we are human. Somehow though we have to fight against this and we need to support families to make the right choices. We need to show people how much a child really needs to eat and we need to do whatever it takes to help get families more active.

The idea of using smaller plates is gathering momentum at various other dietary research organisations. Prof. Jennifer Orlet Fisher is director of the Temple University Center for Obesity Research and Education and its Family Eating Laboratory, and she is one of the world's leading academic authorities on children's nutrition, healthy eating and portion control. She believes that if a child learns now how to stay at a healthy weight through eating the right food and making good lifestyle choices, that child will have a powerful advantage for living a long and healthy life. Prof. Fisher believes that one of the best things a parent can do to help a child get there may be to serve a child's food on small plates.

As you have seen above, Japanese children are served food on smaller plates in reasonable portion sizes for children, with no super-sizing either at home or in restaurants.

Children will self-regulate their food intake when allowed to

In a series of fascinating experiments with hundreds of children from the age of two to 13, Fisher and her colleagues in the food-research community have come to a series of Japanese-style insights, and what she calls 'research-supported, mother-tested strategies' that indicate that smaller portions and smaller plates may give your child a critical health advantage. Children, she has found, when left to their own devices, tend not to serve themselves huge portions. She feels that offering children smaller plates could be helpful in keeping portion size, and appetite, in proper perspective.

Fisher suggests that children be encouraged to select small first portions with additional helpings if they are still hungry and to let children participate in serving themselves. Allow young children to take the lead in deciding how much to eat.

There is a fascinating, preliminary body of more research evidence emerging on the subject of children and serving sizes. Dr Leann Birch and her colleagues noted in a March 2007 paper in the *Journal of Law, Medicine and Ethics* ('Parental influence on eating behaviour: Conception to adolescence') that large food portions promote greater calorie intake by children as young as two years old. They found that when doubling the portion of a main meal dish for preschool-aged children, they ate approximately 25–29 per cent more than would be appropriate for their age, even though they actually consumed only two-thirds of the smaller portions of the dish and were not aware of the increased portion. The authors made an obvious but important point: 'adults, like children, eat more when served large portions'.

Dr Lucy Cooke told us of an interesting effect observed in research: over time, children seem to lose their ability to gauge their appropriate portion sizes. When they are very young they can self-regulate their intake of food, so that if they're given a bigger portion size they stop eating. But by the time they are five that ability seems to have gone. By the age of five they've lost their ability to self-regulate, and they will just eat more because it's there. Cooke says that there is starting to be a feeling among researchers that one of the reasons that formula-fed babies get heavier than breast-fed babies is that they are unintentionally over-fed. The result is that newborn babies can be given portion sizes that are too big for them and this can have a knock-on effect as they grow up. The result is similar when older children are told to finish everything on their plate. A breast-fed baby, in contrast, de-latches when full, and parents don't attempt to make them drink more. The baby is therefore able to self-regulate in a way that a formula-fed baby isn't. It's important for parents to understand that their child can self-regulate. They know how much they need, and you can trust them.

You can read more about feeding in the early years in Appendices I and III.

Cut down on processed foods for the healthiest diet

Although childhood-obesity specialist Dr David L. Katz agrees with the idea of serving foods on modest-sized plates, for him the bigger priority is what foods are on the table. He points out that wholesome, minimally processed foods are self-regulating. They help us to fill up on fewer calories, but for him the crockery used is less of an issue when what's in the dish is good.

Vegetables as a first course

In a Penn State University study of 72 children aged three to five years, researchers found that serving a vegetable soup at the beginning of a meal was an effective way of both boosting a child's vegetable intake and reducing overall calories consumed at the meal. ('Serving large portions of vegetable soup at the start of a meal affected children's energy and vegetable intake', *Appetite*, August 2011.)

In another Penn State University study of 51 children aged three to six years, researchers found that increasing the portion size of vegetables served to preschool children at the start of a meal can lead to increased vegetable consumption. They recommend that childcare providers promote vegetable consumption in young children by serving large portions of vegetables at the start of a meal. ('Eating vegetables first: The use of portion size to increase vegetable intake in preschool children', *American Journal of Clinical Nutrition*, May, 2010.)

According to a 2014 piece in the journal *Appetite* by researcher Roland Sturm of the RAND Corporation, several strategies appear promising for improving portion control for children, including using smaller-diameter and -volume plates, but also reducing total television and other screen watching, and reducing or eliminating eating while watching the television and/or other screens.

Remember that not every day, or every week, is the same

In Australia, dietician Rosemary Stanton told us that the correct portion sizes will vary with the child, and will vary from week to week according to that child's growth pattern. It makes sense, then, to start with a modest portion but to allow the child to request more. This advice does, of course, assume that the family food pattern is high in nutrients, includes more whole grains and plant-based foods and less processed food, added sugars and salt. Stanton added that having more does not include eating junk food, because a child who is having a growth spurt needs more food plus more nutrients. It is also important not to offer junk foods if a child refuses to eat the healthy meal that you have prepared.

Not only does allowing young children to serve themselves at meals mean that they will self-regulate their portions but there are also other developmental benefits as well, including social and motor skills, as was recognised in an April 2013 study published in the journal *Pediatrics* ('Plate size and children's appetite: Effects of larger dishware on self-served portions and intake'); however, it is recognised that children may over-serve themselves if they are given large plates to serve their portions into.

The lessons from Japan: serve a bowl of broth-based clear or vegetable soup during the meal, and serve food on smaller plates – but don't skimp on the fruit and veggies!

Inspire Your Child to Enjoy Daily Physical Activity

Encourage your family to enjoy a minimum of 60
minutes of moderate-intensity physical activity per day.

———————

*Lack of activity destroys the good condition of every
human being while movement and methodical
physical exercise save it and preserve it.*

Plato

Every school day, across the entire nation of Japan, millions of
Japanese children do something that gives them a tremendous
health advantage. It's something that's so easy that you and
your child can begin doing it tomorrow. They walk to school.
And they walk home from school. A lot. Every single school
day. And they do it more than children in most other developed
nations.

A healthy start to each day

That remarkably simple, effective moderate-intensity physical
activity helps them achieve, day in and day out, year after year,
the recommendations of a wide variety of health authorities that
children engage in at least 60 minutes of moderate-to-intense

physical activity every day. They get this dose of physical activity even before any sports time is added. And it may contribute to the fact that Japanese children are projected to enjoy the longest, healthiest lives on earth. Japan is a highly urbanised developed nation, therefore there are many opportunities to walk on safe pavements and back roads.

When I was a girl growing up in Kawasaki, Japan, I and tens of millions of other Japanese children did two things that gave us a powerful health boost. First, we were given 'smart rewards' for doing the daily workout I mentioned earlier, which is organised through a national system called *rajio taiso*, or radio-delivered calisthenics. We participated in a series of exercises in a designated public space near our home every morning at 6.30am over the summer holidays. We were awarded stamps for each day we did the workout. Second, from the age of four until 12, I walked back and forth to school, an average of 2–3 miles in total per day.

Today, years later, when it comes to physical activity, at first glance Japanese children don't seem much different from those in the West. Millions of children go to school every day, where they have break-times and sports, and then they go home to study, do homework, play, watch TV and play video games. But a closer look reveals a big difference, and it confers a huge health advantage. Japanese children enjoy much higher levels of routine incidental exercise built into their daily lives and radically lower levels of commuting in vehicles and school buses. My nephew (aged 17) and niece (15) walk to school for just under ½ mile each way, and another niece (12) for 1 mile.

Today, most Japanese children are performing two key activities: over 75 per cent still take part in the *rajio taiso* system of fun, small, tangible rewards from their schools for daily exercise, and almost 98 per cent of them walk to school. Believe it or not, the network of community support for Japanese children walking to school is so safe, universal and culturally automatic that children as young as seven or eight walk to school without their parents, often in the company of other children, and often looked over by volunteer adults at spots along the way.

In fact, in a well-planned national walking-to-school system of safety and community supervision that has endured since 1953, Japanese children walk an average of about 60 minutes back and forth to school every single school day. On top of this, many Japanese schools give children a series of short physical activity breaks throughout the day, so that they can refocus and recharge.

Thinking back to the past

In the past, I understand that most children in the UK went to their local primary school. The roads weren't so busy, and it was the norm to walk to school where distance wasn't prohibitive. Even today many children can and do walk to school or use the public transport system, which requires walking to the railway or underground station, or bus stop. But things have definitely changed for many families in the UK. Many parents are concerned about allowing their younger children to walk to school without an adult because of busy roads and the fear of abduction. Also, children in the UK today are not guaranteed a place at the school that is closest to them. In those instances they are more likely to have to be driven to school. And for children who live in the countryside, they will almost certainly be getting a school bus or be driven to school.

In Japan, however, the system works differently and the fact that most children walk to school is another public-health triumph. Most Japanese children are meeting the recommendations that children get an average of 60 minutes per day of moderate-to-vigorous physical activity. In fact, Japanese children get 60 minutes per day from walking to school alone, because walking counts as moderate physical activity. Walking is one of the best forms of physical activity because it is easy, efficient and usually doesn't cause injuries.

The importance of play

What about play? Play times at school are opportunities for children to move around, play games and generally let off steam. Of course, as the children get into their teens they may be less likely to want to run about and play sports in their break times. Perhaps as parents, it might be worth thinking about approaching our schools to ask them to give our children more opportunities for physical activity that they might enjoy during break times – I suggest some ways this might be done later in this chapter.

The wisdom of this, and the research to support it, is clear: boys and girls are biologically engineered to move, run and jump, and when they do, they perform better at school, are happier and more focused. And the health benefits of this lifestyle habit may be substantial in helping to give our children the longest, healthiest lives possible.

'Children who walk or bicycle to school have higher daily levels of physical activity and better cardiovascular fitness than do children who do not actively commute to school,' reported Kirsten K Davison, PhD, Jessica L. Werder, MPH, and Catherine T Lawson, PhD in the July 2008 issue of the journal *Preventing Chronic Disease*:

> Despite weak evidence linking active commuting to reduced BMI [body mass index, a measure of a person's weight in relation to their height], research indicates that possible health benefits of active commuting to school include higher rates of physical activity and higher cardiovascular fitness among youth, which are linked with reduced risk for coronary heart disease, stroke, cardiovascular disease, and cancer.

In an article titled 'Walking to school in Japan and childhood obesity prevention: New lessons from an old policy' published in the November 2012 issue of the *American Journal of Public Health*, researchers Nagisa Mori, Francisco Armada and D. Craig Willcox found that Japan has exceptionally high rates (98.3 per cent) of walking or biking to school among children compared with other similar-income countries. The researchers also made a link between this activity and Japan's low levels of childhood obesity.

When American walk-to-school advocate Margo Pedroso returned from a trip to Tokyo, she reported that:

> Parents we met on our trip said walking to school is a basic principle of Japanese life, and that their roads cannot accommodate the traffic that would result from driving to school. They value their children learning how to navigate their neighborhoods and be independent ... Japanese parents are also very concerned about 'stranger danger.' But they manage that fear by near-universal participation in efforts to create 'eyes on the street' and safe routes for children to walk to school. In communities where more parents are working and unavailable, retired adults step up to fill the gap in watching out for children. In Japan, all children are taught safe walking skills at kindergarten, and practice those skills walking to school in groups. In junior school, students learn to take the transit system and navigate other neighborhoods. In the US [and, I would bet, in the UK as well], children would benefit greatly from having bicycle and pedestrian skills built into their curricula. Finally, the Japanese system clearly demonstrates the 'safety in numbers' phenomenon. Because hundreds of children walk to school at the same time, they are very visible to drivers.

The walking school bus

Although Japan might have pioneered the modern age of walking to school over 60 years ago, many developed countries are now promoting walking to school as a tactic to boost physical activity and combat childhood obesity. Across the globe, in places like Auckland, London, Ottawa, Florida, California and Singapore, Walking School Bus programmes, sponsored by governments and schools, are popping up to encourage parents and children to walk to school. It has the beginnings of a beautiful international movement, and I hope it catches on. Scandinavian and Nordic children have been superstars in this field, too: in education-powerhouse Finland, for example, nearly 75 per cent of children walk to school. In New York, when our own son recently turned seven years old, we've been walking part of the way to school with him more and more, and the benefits are fantastic. He gets to school fully awake, refreshed and energised, we have great conversations along the way, and we often run into other children and parents doing the same thing, so it really does turn into a joyful Walking School Bus.

Exercise sets the health and achievement standard for life

According to the American Heart Association, inactive children are likely to become inactive adults. But the good news is that physical activity helps with controlling weight, reducing blood pressure, raising HDL ('good') cholesterol, reducing the risk of diabetes and some kinds of cancer, and improving psychological well-being, including gaining more self-confidence and higher self-esteem.

The World Health Organization also adds that appropriate levels of physical activity for 5–17-year-olds contribute to the development of healthy bones, muscles and joints, as well as a healthy cardiovascular system, coordination and movement control, improving control over symptoms of anxiety and depression, and providing opportunities for a child's self-expression, social interaction and integration.

The benefits to children of regular activity aren't just physical. There are also mental effects that include elevating a child's mood and even boosting performance at school by improving alertness, attention and motivation. They also help to generate new neurological pathways. Researchers at the US Institute of Medicine examined children's exercise programmes and concluded that they help academically. University of Texas epidemiology professor,

Harold Kohl, who led the study of eight- and nine-year-olds, told the *Voice of America* in July 2014:

> The evidence is really emerging in the last five or six years ... Both cognitive studies, brain imaging studies and other [studies] show the acute effects that a bout or two of physical activity has on blood profusion in the brain – in the centers that really help children learn to recall things faster and think faster.

Kohl believes that generally, physically active kids are more likely to achieve their full academic potential versus inactive children. Prof. Charles Hillman at the University of Illinois came to similar conclusions in another recent study ('Effects of the FITKids Randomized Controlled Trial on Executive Control and Brain Function', *Pediatrics*, September 2014), which found that children in the exercise group enjoyed improvements in measurements of both executive function and 'attentional inhibition', the ability to screen out irrelevant information and concentrate on the work at hand.

In 2011 the UK's Chief Medical Officers issued a landmark report titled 'Start Active, Stay Active: A report on physical activity for health from the four home countries', in which they recommended that children under five years old should be encouraged to be active from the early months with floor-based or water-based play in safe environments. When they are ready to move around more, they should be encouraged to play through movement and to avoid being sedentary for extended periods, unless sleeping. All children, from five to 18 years, should aim for moderate- to vigorous-intensity physical activity for at least 60 minutes, and up to several hours every day, and to minimise the amount of time spent sedentary. These recommendations are considered by the UK's top doctors to be essential to benefit the physical and psychological well-being of children and young people.

Fun ways to be more active

Children love to play. It's natural for them and they will find all kinds of ways to play if they are given the opportunity. It's also an excellent way to help them interact with their friends – and it keeps them fit too.

Give young children lots of opportunities to play with their friends, either in the home or outside. If you can, make playing outside in the garden more interesting by giving them boxes to climb into, balls to kick around, inflatable water pools to splash around in in the summer. Check that your school is encouraging active play in the playground, such as skipping, playing chase, hopscotch, or other games that involve running and jumping.

For good, basic all-round exercise, walking is excellent. If you can, as well as walk with your children to school, take them to exercise the dog, walk in the park, the countryside and to the shops.

Moderate-intensity physical activity

All movement is good, but adding in some moderate-intensity exercise is essential too. Moderate-intensity aerobic activity means that you're working hard enough to raise your heart rate and break into a sweat. One way to tell if you're working at a moderate intensity is if you can still talk but you can't sing the words to a song. Encourage your child to ride a scooter or bicycle, or learn how to skateboard or rollerblade. Take your child to an outdoor activity park or adventure playground that has rope ladders, tree houses, walkways and structures to swing on, climb over and wriggle through. Or just step up the walking speed when you go out for your walks together.

Vigorous-intensity physical activity

Getting some vigorous-intensity activity is also essential. This kind of exercise makes you breathe hard and fast, and your heart rate will have gone up quite a bit. If you're working at this level, you won't be able to say more than a few words without pausing for a breath. Apart from obvious choices such as playing a sport – football, youth rugby, tennis, badminton or netball – there are other forms of exercise that might appeal to children and young people who are not quite so sporty. Many children enjoy splashing about at the swimming pool and learning to swim. They might also like to join a traditional ballet class or a modern dance class, or take up running, or a martial art, such as karate. You can also find gym classes for pre-school children, which can be great fun.

Muscle-building exercise

All kinds of traditional games that children have played in the past can be good exercise and help to build strength and improve coordination. For young people, muscle-strengthening activities are those that require them to lift their own body weight or to work against a resistance, such as climbing a rope. Once children get a bit older they will often enjoy tug of war, swinging on playground equipment bars, gymnastics, rope or tree climbing and indoor climbing, but many of the sports and activities listed earlier will also build muscle and improve coordination as well.

Making changes

In many parts of the world it's just not practical for children to walk to school by themselves in the same way that Japanese children do, at least not yet. But perhaps you can try walking with your child at least part of the way to school on some days of the week. You could also perhaps organise a Walk to School Programme in your local area. You could also experiment with encouraging your child to enjoy different combinations of the many activities above, to increase his or her activity levels.

Moving about should be a necessity in life – it isn't so much for most of us these days, so we have to make it more so. Schools could do a lot more to encourage physical activity that is purely fun. Not every child likes organised sports, but they might enjoy more active free-play in the playground, or dancing or aerobics classes that don't require specialised sports ability.

Perhaps we should ask our schools to allow a long skipping rope to be taken into school. It's what many children did in the past at primary school and all the girls skipped in a long line. A return to traditional games could be fun, but many are banned by schools because of the fear that a child will fall and hurt themselves. Perhaps parents and schools could relax a little and consider the benefits of more physical activity versus the risk of an occasional skinned knee! When I went to primary school in Japan, break-time and after-school activity was open-ended, outdoor, free physical play, either in the school's open field equipped with climbing poles, horizontal bars and jungle gyms, or in playgrounds, or the little hills and fields near our home.

Children today should be encouraged to take more unstructured free-play indoors and outdoors, where they can choose the activity they enjoy the most. What we need to do as adults is make sure they have safe spaces to play in.

Your example counts

It's obviously important for adults to be a role model to their children for physical activity. As Yoni Freedhoff, MD, assistant professor of family medicine at the University of Ottawa, notes, 'any parent who wants their children to be regularly physically active needs to be regularly physically active too'. Australian dietician Rosemary Stanton also points out that physical activity as a family – such as going for walks, playing sports, swimming or dancing – strengthens family ties. And Dr David Katz of Yale University Medical School emphasises the fun aspect of physical activity, 'Health should not be such a chore. It's a prize!' (You can read more about being a role model in Appendix II.)

In our own family, we decided a few years ago to mostly unplug all screens at home, and to trade that time for outdoor free-play in a local playground, for family sports such as running,

Frisbee, ball-playing and power-walking. We also participate in local volunteer projects such as mulching and planting young trees, often in New York's Central Park, which we are lucky to live close to. Our son, now seven years old, enjoys taking part in all these activities with us.

We also often explore the city on foot. One day on the way to a classmate's birthday party some way from our home, our son suggested that, instead of taking a bus after we got off the subway, we walk part of the way on the High Line. This remarkable urban redevelopment is a linear public park, about 1½ miles long, built on an elevated, unused freight railway. What a pleasure it was to walk on that urban-nature trail. One summer evening, after a fun-filled day in the newly developed, gorgeous Brooklyn River Park, where we had played in a water playground and sand playground, and dipped our toes in a mini-beach on the East River, our son said, 'Let's walk across the Brooklyn Bridge [just over a mile long] back to Manhattan.' On the spur of the moment, that's what we did. We walked into the sun setting in the downtown skyline, with breezes running through our hair, as the East River churned beneath us. It was a sublime, unexpected experience – and all we did was walk!

I think this just shows that walking and getting outside can be fun, even in big cities. And today in the UK there are play areas and parks in most localities.

Living a largely 'unplugged' life at home and after work and school hours has been much easier that we thought. And it is infinitely more fun, engaging and exhilarating than staring at electronic screens.

Make regular physical activity and exercise a family mission that you love. Get moving, every day, have fun and enjoy it!

Nurture a Wrap-around Family Lifestyle

Create a wrap-around home environment that supports healthy food and lifestyle choices. Eat family meals together as a regular practice. Practise healthy, delicious cooking and eating as an example for your children.

———————

To bed early, wake up early, eat breakfast as a family.
Food tastes best when the family eats together.
Japanese *Shokuiku* food education slogans

In Japan, it's pretty easy for a child to enjoy a healthy lifestyle. As I discussed in previous chapters, the foods they eat at home and elsewhere are presented in an overall pattern that is lower in empty calories, higher in nutrients and more efficiently filling than the patterns that have often become routine in other developed nations. Portion sizes are smaller, and desserts are much smaller and less frequent. Most Japanese children walk to school every day, giving them a major physical activity boost, even before they participate in sports.

The whole Japanese culture, even though it has been highly modernised and Westernised, still provides a national social structure that largely supports and guides children towards healthy behaviour. But I totally understand that in much of the rest of the world, it can be much more difficult for children to be healthy. In the UK, the US and other parts of the world, the media bombards children with advertising for unhealthy food choices at fast food restaurants and supermarkets, where large portions are showcased. Living in New York, we face the same challenges that you may face.

A solution to the unhealthy pressures on today's kids

Children's eating routines can be victimised by overwhelming amounts of high-calorie junk food, fizzy drinks and added sugar on offer. In many places, there are no safe pavements or routes for children to walk or bike to school. The time children might find for enjoyable physical activity is gobbled up by schoolwork or screen time, which happens in Japan, too. Tethered to their smartphones and packed schedules, parents and children feel over-stressed and pressed for time, leaving no room for healthier choices.

There is, however, an amazing Japanese secret for nurturing healthy children that almost every single school-aged child in Japan enjoys. It is a secret that may be a critical contributor towards Japan's number-1 spot in the World Health Olympics of healthy longevity. It makes healthy eating, and cleaning up, a communal, cooperative, pleasurable, educational routine that is practically built into a child's DNA. And it offers a lesson that you can put into action at home for your own child's good health, starting today.

It is the concept of giving your child a wrap-around lifestyle inspired by healthy food choices. It is a series of insights that is rooted in traditional Japanese food practices, but it is also reflected in the cutting-edge, research-based recommendations of many of the world's leading experts for improving children's health.

School meals with a difference

In Japan, millions of children enjoy lunch at their schools every single school day. It is called *gakko kyushoku*, and it includes more than just the meal itself. In a remarkable, universal national programme in the state-run schools that started 60 years ago, Japanese children from elementary school age are required to be:

- Given a fixed choice of very healthy foods and dishes at lunch. These are often fresh and locally grown.

- Taught about the foods and how they are grown – many students are encouraged to visit local farms through grass-roots food education initiatives.

- Help prepare, carry and take turns serving the food to each other.

- Eat as a group with each other and with their adults at a fixed time every day.

- Help clean up the dishes and tables.

Japanese schools turn children into healthy foodies by involving them directly in the process of preparing and serving healthy food as an automatic daily routine. They also narrow the choices available to only delicious, healthy options (which include traditional Japanese meals as well as introductions to other world cuisines), not the buffet-style, 'free choice' approach common to schools in many other nations. Through the school year, a child might experience global dishes such as Korean bibimbap (rice topped with seasoned meat and vegetables), tandoori chicken, spaghetti pescatore and minestrone soup. Unhealthy food options and patterns are simply excluded from the environment for the seven or eight hours a day the child spends in school, and replaced with a gold-standard approach, supported by school-based nutritionists. Some 94 per cent of all public elementary and middle schools in Japan take part in the school lunch programme.

When I was a girl in school in Japan, I was a part of this

system called *kyushoku toban*, or 'staff lunch'. From the age of six onwards, every day a small group of students was assigned to a 'lunch job'. The students took turns putting on chef's hats and smocks, going to the school kitchen to receive from the chefs and kitchen workers two or three big pots of lunch, cartons of beverages, individual trays, plates, bowls and utensils for the class, and serving each other a nutritious hot lunch in the classroom, not a cafeteria. Then we helped each other clean up after the meal, including bringing used tableware, cups, pots and utensils back to the kitchen and wiping the desks. 'We Japanese call it "eating from the same bowl",' explains school principal Kimiko Koyasu. 'No matter how old you are, you never forget what you ate back in school.'

Balanced meals based on a traditional cuisine

The nationwide school lunch programme was originally intended as food for hungry children in the wake of Japan's post-war economic devastation. After 2004, as Japanese eating habits declined and problems of eating disorders, childhood obesity, breakfast-skipping and over-indulgence in fast food emerged in Japan, the emphasis changed and a national law was passed requiring *Shokuiku*, or food education, in schools. Now, according to a 2013 *Washington Post* article by Chico Harlan and Yuki Oda, 'Schools in Japan give their students the sort of food they'd get at home ... The meals are often made from scratch. They're balanced but hearty, heavy on rice and vegetables, fish and soups, and they haven't changed much in four decades.' The choices are extremely narrow: 'They get identical meals, and if they leave food untouched, they are out of luck: Their schools have no vending machines.'

The premium restaurant-quality school food is made largely from scratch from locally produced ingredients and with only small amounts of fried foods and few desserts other than fruit or yoghurt. It is so good, according to Tatsuji Shino, principal at Umejima Elementary School in Tokyo, that parents hear their children talking about what they had for lunch, and the children ask their parents to re-create the meals at home. Some parents ask the schools to share their recipes with them. For Japanese remembering their childhood, the memory of *gakko-kyushoku* conjures up such powerful nostalgia for days of youthful cooperation and friendship that some restaurants offer *kyushoku* menus.

Food education is now a big part of Japan's amazing school lunch programme. It teaches an appreciation of nature that brings us all the wonderful foods, and an appreciation of the people who grow, produce and cook them, as well as an understanding of nutrition, health, cooking, table manners, cooperation and social skills, and it encourages children towards a path of healthy lifetime habits. Guest lecturers such as farmers, food specialists and parents are invited to speak to children. Students are taught lessons such as, 'Avoid buying food from convenience stores', 'Choose a traditional Japanese meal over fast food' and 'Early to bed, early to rise, no skipping breakfast.'

The focus on not skipping breakfast is considered very important. According to the 2010 Japanese Government's National Academic Scholarly Learning Ability Survey of 11- and 12-year-olds there was a significant association between eating breakfast and better academic performance on language and maths tests.

An education in working and food production

The children also learn about the fishing, farming and food production industries and about seasonal food festivals, cultivating vegetables, food history, local farmers and home-town food specialities. They learn about the wisdom of the traditional Japanese meal pattern known as *ichiju-sansai*: one soup, three dishes (as explained in Part 3 Chapter 1). Many schools have little gardens where children help to grow some of the food that's eaten.

A Canadian journalist named Danielle Nerman recently toured Japanese schools and witnessed Japan's wrap-around school approach in action:

At Sanya Elementary in the Tokyo suburb of Suginami, I watched a group of students haul heavy trays of service dishes and pots of hot food into their classroom. Wearing matching white chef's hats and sanitary masks, they quickly and confidently ladle steaming miso into bowls for their teachers and classmates. There is no room here for picky eaters. Everyone gets the same lunch and eats together, at their desks. [Then] a small girl stood up and began what is a daily ritual at Sanya Elementary. She read the entire lunch menu out loud to her classmates. After the meal, students drew pictures of the ingredients they just ate and stuck them to a map of Japan on the wall. Images of plump purple grapes and pieces of ginger were strategically placed in the region they were grown to illustrate the importance of local produce. (CBS News, 12 January 2015)

'What is most difficult for me to explain is why we can do this and other countries cannot,' wondered Masahiro Oji, a government director of school health education. 'Japan's standpoint is that school lunches are a part of education, not a break from it.'

A culinary dream come true

One day, not long ago in Tokyo, a nutritionist and mother named Tsuguko Matsumoto remembered a dream she had when her daughter was a small child and she was struggling to balance work and family.

In the dream, which she recounted in the Japanese government nutrition report 'Shokuiku Textbook for Parents and Children', Ms Matsumoto came home from work one night to the beautiful sight of her young daughter wearing an apron and saying, 'Mum, welcome home! I made dinner!' When she awoke, she wondered, 'How will I realise this dream?' How could she instil in her daughter, now a toddler, a love and respect for preparing healthy food that would stay with her until adulthood?

Then and there, Ms Matsumoto decided she would try to make her dream come true. The first thing she did was make her child a 'partner in the kitchen'. Every night, she recalled, 'I let my child play in a corner of the kitchen, where I could see her and could always talk to her. When she started crawling, she moved to the area below the sink, took pots and bowls out and played with them, banging on them with a whisk. She didn't care much for toys but loved to play with the kitchen utensils!

'Once she learned to stand, I let her stand on a footstool and play with water in the sink. She enjoyed rinsing vegetables and tearing them. When she was a bit older, I let her use a knife. First, a fruit knife: I let her cut a cucumber and potato. I had to keep my eyes on her at the beginning and it took a long time to prepare a meal. She gained skill and she surprised me with her rapid mastery of use of knives without having a major injury.' She added, 'While I let my child stand in the kitchen with me, rather than considering her an obstacle for housework, she gradually became my good partner.'

Soon, she remembered, 'We got into the groove of baking during weekends. We used simple recipes that required measuring ingredients, mixing and baking. We spread newspapers all over the kitchen floor, played a Disney tune, and we were ready to start. Sometimes, knowing that I couldn't do it well, I despaired. But my child's expressions of delight and joy saved me.'

Ms Matsumoto took some of the baked goods to her office the next day, and they were so tasty that her colleagues wrote thank you messages to the girl saying 'Gochiso-sama' ('That was a feast!'). The little girl was so excited that she declared, 'I'm going to bake again!'

Then, one day during a summer break when her daughter was 13, Ms Matsumoto's dream came true.

'Mum, welcome home!' said the child, 'I made dinner!'

Later, her class had a lesson on growing vegetables. Ms Matsumoto's parents, who were rural farmers, agreed to help out. Ms Matsumoto recalled, 'They sent the class vegetables enough for all the students, and individual pictures of farming equipment and every kind of vegetable they harvested, like pumpkin, aubergine and sesame.' In response, the schoolchildren sent back a booklet of student essays thanking them for the food education.

A few years ago, Ms Matsumoto's mother posted the booklet to her granddaughter, with a note that said, 'I reread these essays for the first time in years. I was once again moved by the words filled with the children's honest appreciation. I thank my granddaughter for this indispensable experience. I'd like to take the booklet with me to the other world, so please be sure to return it to me.'

Today, reports Ms Matsumoto, 'My daughter made my dream come true. She has acquired real tastes and skills. Her motto is "Fun to cook, delicious to eat and happy to serve." Now she is in high school. Her favourite class is cooking. She is cooking the cuisines of the world and she has tried more than 40 recipes in the last two years. She brings baked goods to school, a snack to an after-school teacher, and she entertains her friends with home-cooked meals at home. She has grown into a daughter who is so much more than I dreamed of.'

Reflecting on her 17 years of food education as a parent, Ms Matsumoto realised that the Chinese character 'food' is written as 'making a good person'. She marvelled that 'My daughter learned to give joy to others through food. I thank her.'

It all started with a dream, and an invitation to a two-year-old to play in a corner of the kitchen.

> Ms Matsumoto and her daughter, along with millions of children in thousands of Japanese schools, have discovered a global insight that can inspire children and parents anywhere in the world: children will eat healthy delicious food if you start them early and give them a wrap-around environment that celebrates healthy choices.

The importance of being involved

The idea of bringing children into the kitchen as a pathway to health was recently supported by a study of a group of six- to ten-year-old children published in the August 2014 journal *Appetite* ('Involving children in meal preparation: Effects on food intake'). The researchers concluded that when you involve children in meal preparation it can increase the amount of vegetables they eat. The study also says that encouraging parents to involve their children in the preparation of healthy and balanced meals could be a valuable intervention strategy to improve children's diets.

The idea of eating family meals together is a practice that many families around the world, including in Japan, are finding harder and harder to pull off, as parents work later and after-school schedules get over-stressed. But it is a goal worth heroically striving for, because the potential health benefits for children appear to be huge. Here are just a few examples:

- A research paper published in the November 2014 issue of *Pediatrics* ('Childhood Obesity and Interpersonal Dynamics During Family Meals') reported that warmth, group enjoyment and parental positive reinforcement at family meals were significantly associated with reduced risk of childhood overweight and obesity.

- According to the Center for Families at Purdue University, surveys indicate that 80 per cent of families value meal-times together, but only 33 per cent successfully achieve daily family meals. They found that the quality of food is higher where family meals are taken, plus there is less over-weight, enhanced language skills and academic performance, improved social skills and family unity, and a reduction in risk-taking behaviours.

- Improved achievement test scores: A University of Illinois study of 120 boys and girls aged seven to 11 found that children who did well in school and on achievement tests were those who generally spent large amounts of time eating meals with their families.

- Higher school achievement: research by the National Center on Addiction and Substance Abuse at Columbia University (CASA), and others, has found a strong relationship between the frequency of family meals and school achievement scores.

- Reduced likelihood of smoking, drinking, or taking drugs: in a research project coordinated by Dr Blake Bowden of Cincinnati Children's Hospital, 527 teenagers were studied to determine which family and lifestyle characteristics were related to good mental health and adjustment. He found that kids who ate dinner with their families at least five times per week were the least likely to take drugs, feel depressed or get into trouble.

- According to CASA surveys, teens who eat dinner with their parents twice a week or less are four times more likely to smoke cigarettes, three times more likely to smoke marijuana, and nearly twice as likely to drink as those who eat dinner with their parents six or seven times a week. Teens who eat frequent family dinners are also less likely than other teens to have sex at young ages or to get into fights; they are at lower risk for thoughts of suicide and are likelier to do better in school. This is true regardless of a teen's gender, family structure, or family socioeconomic level. Teens who have frequent family dinners are more likely to be emotionally content, work hard at school and have positive peer relationships, not to mention healthier eating habits.

- Dianne Neumark-Sztainer and her colleagues at the University of Minnesota published the results of the EAT study (which stands for 'eating among teens') in the *Journal of the American Dietetic Association*. Their findings showed a dramatic relationship between family meal patterns and dietary intake in adolescents. Their study involved nearly 5,000 students of diverse ethnic and socio-economic backgrounds. They found that family meals were associated with improved intakes of fruits, vegetables, grains, calcium-rich foods, protein, iron, fibre and vitamins A, C, E, B_6 and folate. Family meals were associated with a lower intake of soft drinks and snack foods. The Project EAT survey also found that girls who ate more frequent family meals exhibited less 'disordered eating', including dieting behaviours, extreme weight control behaviours, binge eating and chronic dieting.

'Ultimately, what we as parents must do is live the lives we want our children to live,' said Dr Yoni Freedhoff. He told us, 'Health-wise, that would include reclaiming the kitchen as an important and beloved room in our homes and ensure that it's used regularly, not just for the assembly of ready-made ingredients, but in the actual transformation of whole ingredients into meals, and also in ensuring that our children don't leave home knowing how to play soccer, but not knowing how to cook.'

Reduce television watching for good health

There is one more idea for a healthy 'wrap-around' home environment that many experts agree on: minimise children's screen time, especially TV.

A January 2013 study by the Pennington Biomedical Research Center in the US titled 'Television, adiposity and cardiometabolic risk in children', and published in the *American Journal of Preventive Medicine,* found that having a TV in the bedroom has a bigger negative impact on children's health, including weight, than earlier believed. A television in the bedroom, it appears, can disrupt healthy habits, leading to lower amounts of sleep and eating meals with the family less often, which in turn can lead to weight gain and obesity.

According to a June 2012 report in the journal *Physiology and Behavior* ('ObesiTV: How television is influencing the obesity epidemic'), there is growing evidence that television viewing is a major contributor to the obesity epidemic, and the authors of the paper found indications of a direct association between time spent watching television and body weight. Possible reasons for the relationship include: TV acting as a sedentary replacement for physical activity; TV food ads stimulating intake of less healthy foods; TV fuelling 'mindless' eating; and TV programmes that present cooking, eating and rapid weight loss as entertainment.

How can you adopt a wrap-around family lifestyle?

What are the lessons you can learn from Japanese schools and homes, and from the insights of global health researchers?

You probably can't strongly influence what your child eats at school, birthday parties and play dates, but you can build a powerful, Japanese-style zone of healthy behaviours, choices and treats in your home. You can do this through your own behaviour and by de-cluttering and streamlining your kitchen and home environment of unhealthy patterns, including consuming fewer unhealthy foods and avoiding excessive screen time. And if you start these practices early, your child can learn to make healthy choices on his or her own.

You probably can't change your child's school lunch programme to reflect the Japanese system, but you can apply the same insights to your own child's home environment to help nurture a wrap-around lifestyle. If you offer your child a fixed choice of healthy foods, discuss where the foods come from, how and where they grow, take them to local markets, involve them in the food preparation process, eat with them every day, and minimise the availability of less healthy options in your home, you'll be following some of the best advice from experts on child health and nutrition. (Remember: be careful with all knives, of course, especially sharp ones, but children can also help separate, wash, chop and prepare some foods with blunt knives or special children's kitchenware, as well as measuring ingredients, stirring and mixing, which many children love to do.)

You can also visit local farms as a family weekend excursion. William and I have taken our son to an egg-collecting event at the famed Stone Barns Farm in Pocantico Hills, and to a spring sheep-shearing demonstration at the Queens County Farm, the oldest working farm in New York State. One of my dreams is to send our son to his paternal great-grandparents' working farm, for an extended period of time, for hands-on experience as a rice-paddy farmer. Many farms and botanic garden museums offer one-day volunteer opportunities and/or school-age children camps. In the UK, for example, NamaYasai Farm in Lewes, Sussex, grows Japanese vegetables and welcomes anybody, regardless of age, to visit and help out.

We have had cooking playdates for our son and his friends and hands-on cooking sessions at his pre-school. We explained where some of the ingredients like rice grains and kombu sea vegetables came from, and showed harvesting photos. We chose for our sessions to make vegetable (avocado and carrot) *makizushi*, roll-sushi and *oshizush*, or pressed-sushi, because we thought that the children would enjoy the process of slicing avocado and carrots, layering the ingredients, rolling and pressing them in sushi moulds and, of course, serving and eating them. The children had loads of fun.

Children naturally love to help prepare meals, and it's a wonderful way not only to learn to eat well but also to use various skills in an enjoyable way, such as reading (the recipe), following steps (the recipe), maths (counting and measuring the ingredients), science (basic food chemistry, agriculture, ocean science, climate, the seasons), culture, art (serving and decorating) and to help develop hand–eye coordination (for measuring, mixing, cutting and shaping).

A child's healthy eating – in a nutshell

This expert opinion comes from Dr Lucy Cooke, CPsychol, Senior Research Psychologist, Health Behaviour Research Centre University College London.

There is evidence that food preferences and eating behaviour are partly inherited, but there is a lot that parents can do to improve things:

- Act as a role model for healthy eating.
- Offer disliked (usually healthy) foods in small quantities frequently and repeatedly.
- Offer fruit and vegetables as snacks.
- Keep unhealthy foods and drinks out of the house.
- Eat together with children.
- Let children help to prepare foods and choose them in the supermarket.
- Offer choices, but only between healthy foods.
- Don't use food as a reward.

The lesson of healthy wrap-around Japanese food and lifestyle patterns is not that your family needs to eat Japanese food to be healthy. The lesson is that you can think of many Japanese food and lifestyle habits as reflections of the wisdom of the world's best experts – including our very own parents and ancestors who had healthier and more traditional lifestyles – and reminders of wisdom to help inspire our children to live long and healthy lives.

Be Your Child's
Lifestyle Authority

Communicate food and lifestyle habits to your children
in an authoritative rather than an authoritarian style.

---

*Send the beloved children on a journey – to gain
strength, wisdom and experience.*

Japanese saying

There is a final promise that Japan offers us, and there is a final
insight that gives us hope of making the promise come true, to
help us guide our children towards a lifelong journey of good
health. The promise of Japan is that it is possible for us as parents,
anywhere in the world, to build an environment for children that,
although far from perfect, can inspire them towards adopting
tastes and habits that will increase their chances of enjoying as
long and healthy a life as it's possible for them to experience.

The insight is for us to be our children's example, leader,
model and authority by communicating lifestyle habits to them
in an authoritative style.

The lesson of the 'World's Healthiest Children' is not that
there is anything inherently Japanese about healthy longevity,
nor is there anything inherently better or more enlightened
about Japanese children, Japanese parents or Japanese foods.

The world-topping healthy longevity projected for Japanese children today is instead a reflection of a larger pattern of behaviours, in action, that can help the health of children anywhere in the world thrive and flourish. Japan came upon this pattern almost accidentally, largely as a product of its available geography, climate and resources, cumulative wisdom passed down from generation to generation, and some smart public policies, and it has tried to adhere to the pattern for a pragmatic, common-sense reason: it works. When combined with a superb national health-care system, the practices of relatively healthy eating and physical activity patterns enjoyed by the Japanese have helped their nation to consistently achieve world-leading longevity and healthy longevity rankings for several decades.

For the rest of us who don't live in Japan, however, how can we apply these insights to help our children have a healthy life? It turns out that there is one parenting style that might be a great help.

The authoritative parent

Every child is different and every parent is different, and what works for one may not work for another, especially when different cultures and traditions are factored into the equation. But it looks as though, based on the evidence, for many parents an *authoritative style* is an excellent choice. It is a style of parenting that is endorsed by a very wide variety of childhood development experts, and it appears to have a sharp health payoff for children.

The idea of authoritative parenting was pioneered in the early 1960s by the psychologist Diana Baumrind. Her research identified three styles of parenting: authoritarian, authoritative and permissive parenting.

In the authoritarian style, parents set strict rules without explaining the reasons for them. Such parents are focused on family status, unquestioning obedience, power and coercion, and are not responsive to their children. She observed that children of authoritarian parents tended to be obedient, but lower in happiness, social competence and self-esteem.

Authoritative parents, by contrast, also establish guidelines and rules that their children are expected to follow, but the big difference is that these parents are responsive, willing to listen to questions and are more nurturing and strategic in their approach to discipline. Authoritative parents monitor and communicate clear standards for their children's conduct. They are assertive, but not intrusive and restrictive. Their disciplinary methods are supportive, rather than punitive. They want their children to be assertive as well as socially responsible, and self-regulated as well as cooperative. 'The authoritative model of discipline', Baumrind wrote, 'is characterised by the use of firm control contingently applied and justified by rational explanation of consistently enforced rules.'

The benefits of the authoritative approach

Baumrind and other researchers have observed that the children of authoritative parents tend to be happier, more self-confident about their abilities to learn new skills, more socially adept, and have better emotional control, self-regulation and academic achievement. Here are some of the things authoritative parents tend to do:

- Place high expectations and consistent boundaries on their children's behaviour.

- Listen to their children, and allow them to ask questions and express opinions.

- Guide their children in a rational, issue-oriented way by explaining the reasoning behind the rules.

- Serve as a role model for the behaviours they expect from their children.

- Are warm and nurturing, and consistent and fair with discipline.

- Foster self-confidence by expecting children to use reason and independence, allowing them to make mistakes and learn from them, and expecting a child to achieve self-regulation.

- Establish what Baumrind calls a warm, engaged rational parent-child relationship.

The point of authoritative parenting is to guide children to take good decisions, forming good habits and behaviours on their own initiative. Nancy Darling PhD of Oberlin College in Ohio has explained that authoritative parents teach and guide their children, and in doing so they socialise them to accept and value the parents' values. The word 'authoritative' was chosen to imply that parents have power because they are wiser and are legitimate guides to the culture. Prof. Darling notes that authoritative parents set fewer rules but they are better at enforcing them.

The health rewards from authoritative parenting

A wide variety of research studies show that the authoritative parenting style has been associated with healthy lifestyle habits for children.

As Dr Joseph Arnold Skelton, MD, and his colleagues wrote in the December 2011 issue of *Pediatric Clinics of North America*:

Authoritarian parenting styles, characterized by restriction, pressures to eat certain foods, and over-monitoring, are most consistently linked to pediatric weight gain. However, children raised by authoritative parents who promote responsibility, monitoring, and modeling, are more likely to have healthier nutrition and lower BMIs. Child-centred feeding practices, positive nutrition encouragement, and parents' intake of fruits and vegetables are also positively associated with fruit and vegetable consumption in their children.

Here are some of the other observations and suggested findings that researchers have reported:

- An authoritative parenting style can provide the structure and support needed for family meals to occur.
- Children raised in authoritative homes ate more healthily, were more physically active and had lower BMI levels, compared to children who were raised using other styles.
- An authoritative parenting style provides structure, and children tend to exhibit positive behaviour, including eating well, compared to those parented using other styles such as authoritarian, permissive and neglectful parenting.
- Adolescents raised by authoritative parents have better home, health and emotional adjustment compared to adolescents raised by authoritarian parents.
- Authoritative parents give positive feedback, encouragement and physical affection and this has predicted a lower risk of stress, tension, fatigue and risky behaviours of adolescents.
- Obesity is more highly associated with the authoritarian parenting style.
- Use of authoritative feeding practices can reduce the risk of obesity in children.

In Japan, I'm sure there are plenty of parents who follow other parenting styles, and mums and dads who are over-indulgent or authoritarian, but the authoritative style is most in line with what I've noticed to be typical when it comes to children's food and lifestyle habits in Japan.

The division of responsibility

A vivid example of an authoritative parent in action is in one widely respected approach to the complex and critical issue of child feeding. Ellyn Satter is a grandmother, psychotherapist, child nutrition authority and registered dietician based in Wisconsin. She has developed an approach to child feeding called 'The Division of Responsibility', which is rooted in the concept of authoritative parenting. It is an approach that is very widely hailed by many experts for offering children the possibility of establishing lifelong healthy eating habits. Simply stated, Satter explains the concept: 'Parents are responsible for what food they serve to their children, and when and where they serve it; children are responsible for how much of that food they eat and whether they eat any of it at all.'

I see major parallels between Satter's approach and the patterns of Japanese attitudes and practices that have nurtured the world's healthiest children. Satter believes that parents should be the leaders and role models, they should be flexible within firm guidelines, they should invite children into the experience of preparing and enjoying regular family meals, they should regularly expose children to both healthy choices and treats, and that they should neither over-indulge nor over-pressure children when it comes to eating. Once the child is ready for family foods, there should be no special 'kiddie meals' and no forbidden foods, with no forcing children to clean their plate or eat their vegetables. Satter explains that 'Parents must not pin their hopes or their feelings of success on getting the food in the child. They need to remember they have control over what they put on the table. Over whether the child eats it, they do not have control.'

An authoritarian parent, for example, might say, 'Here is your food. Eat it.' A permissive parent would say: 'What would you like? When would you like it?' But an authoritative parent would say, 'Here is what we have to eat. You may eat it or not. You may eat again at snack time.' Or, 'Here's tonight's dinner. I hope you can find something to enjoy.' Here, Satter explains the approach in detail.

'The division of responsibility in feeding' by Ellyn Satter

Raise a healthy child who is a joy to feed

Focus on how you feed and how your child feels and behaves at mealtimes, not on what your child eats. Follow the division of responsibility in feeding. When you maintain the quality of your feeding relationship rather than worrying about what or how much your child eats, your child will eat and grow well and, sooner or later, he will learn to eat almost everything you eat. In the meantime, understand and expect normal child eating behaviour. Your child is likely to be a picky eater, to eat only one or two foods from any meal, to eat a food one time and ignore it another, to eat a lot one time and not much another, and to not eat vegetables.

Your child is a competent eater when:

- He feels good about eating. He enjoys food and joins in happily with family meals and snacks.

- He enjoys meals and behaves nicely at mealtime. He feels good about being included in family meals and does his part to make mealtimes pleasant. He does not make a fuss.

- He picks and chooses from food you make available. He is OK with being offered food he has never seen before. He says 'yes, please,' and 'no, thank you'.

- He ignores food he does not want and also 'sneaks up' on new food and learns to like it. Eventually he will learn to eat almost everything you do.

- He determines for himself how much to eat. Only he knows how much that is. Trusting him to eat as

➡

much as he needs lets him grow consistently and develop the body that nature intended for him.

- Children have natural ability with eating. They eat as much as they need, they grow in the way that is right for them, and they learn to eat the food their parents eat. Step-by-step, throughout their growing-up years, they build on their natural ability and become eating competent. Parents let them learn and grow with eating when they follow the Division of Responsibility in Feeding.

The division of responsibility for infants:

- The parent is responsible for what the child eats.
- The child is responsible for how much he eats (and for everything else).
- Parents choose breast- or formula-feeding, and help the infant to be calm and organised. Then they feed smoothly, paying attention to information coming from the baby about timing, tempo, frequency and amounts.

The division of responsibility for infants making the transition to family food:

- The parent is still responsible for what, and is becoming responsible for when and where the child is fed.
- The child is still and always will be responsible for how much and whether to eat the foods offered by the parent.
- Based on what the child can do, not on how old he is, parents guide the child's transition from nipple feeding through semi-solids, then thick-and-lumpy food, to finger food at family meals.

The division of responsibility for toddlers and adolescents:

- The parent is responsible for what, when, where.

- The child is responsible for how much and whether.

- Fundamental to parents' jobs is trusting children to determine how much and whether to eat from what the parents provide. When parents do their jobs with feeding, children do their jobs with eating:

Parents' feeding jobs:

- Choose and prepare the food.

- Provide regular meals and snacks.

- Make eating times pleasant.

- Step-by-step, show children by example how to behave at family mealtimes.

- Be considerate of children's lack of food experience without catering to likes and dislikes.

- Not let children have food or beverages (except for water) between meal and snack times.

- Let children grow up to get bodies that are right for them.

Children's eating jobs:

- Children will eat.

- They will eat the amount they need.

- They will learn to eat the food their parents eat.

- They will grow predictably.

- They will learn to behave well at mealtimes.

(See more at: http://ellynsatterinstitute.org Reproduced by permission of Ellyn Satter.)

The approach works in Japanese culture

This pattern of the 'Division of Responsibility', it turns out, fits the way Japanese traditionally eat and serve family meals, especially in multi-generation family households. Taking family members' food preferences into consideration, a meal preparer (often a mother), prepares a wide variety of dishes, not one big portion of one or two dishes, and serves them in a communal style. Some members eat more of their favourite dishes and less of their not-so-favourite dishes. Everyone has some foods that he or she likes to eat and is content.

When a child in the family does not want to eat or even try a particular dish, as often happens, a parent gently encourages the child to try the dish. She doesn't. But as she watches other members eat it, after a few meal occasions, and after gentle, positive suggestions, and natural exposure to the same dish, one day, the child decides to try it. She tries a small bite, and guess what? She doesn't hate it!

For example, the mother serves rice, miso soup with wakame sea vegetables and chopped spring onions, pan-grilled mackerel, simmered seasonal vegetables, tofu, sweet miso-flavoured grilled aubergines, ginger stir-fried pork slices, onions and cabbages, and some picked cucumbers. The father loves mackerel and simmered seasonal vegetables, so he eats more of them, and good portions of the other dishes. The grandfather loves tofu and aubergines, so eats more of them and good portions of the other dishes. The older son and the mother like everything and eat even portions of each dish. The younger daughter does not like mackerel, so she doesn't touch it. The grandpa says to her, 'Why don't you have some mackerel. It is in season! It's juicy and meltingly tender.' She doesn't want to try. She enjoys other dishes and everyone is happy and content. Then, mackerel, cooked in different ways, is served time and again, while it's in season, along with a variety of dishes. The family members, especially the father, enjoy it tremendously. After repeated exposures, gentle nudges (no pressure) by the grandpa, dad and mum alternately, everyone seems to enjoy the fish, and the fact that her father looks so happy and brims with the joy of eating mackerel every single time he brings a piece to his mouth, the daughter starts to feel that maybe she'd try a little bit. And one day she does.

To me, this is a vivid illustration of the practice of example-setting, and authoritative parenting – the parent decides what to serve and the child decides what to eat.

Whatever path your family takes, we wish you and your children a long life of joy, wisdom, discovery, compassion, great food and lots of physical activity as you journey through life together. In the words of an old Japanese saying:

'To have children is the fulfilment of all things.'

The Seven Secrets to Nurture Your Child's Health

1: Tweak Your Family Meals

Enjoy family meals that are higher in nutrients, include more plant-based foods and whole grains, and contain less processed food, added sugars and salt.

2: Celebrate Food Joy and Flexible Restraint

Practise flexible restraint, not severe food restriction or food demonization; make eating joyful.

3: Inspire Your Child to Enjoy New Foods

Gently encourage your child to try to enjoy a wide variety of different healthy foods, including many different fruits and vegetables.

4: Rebalance The Family Plate – With Japanese-style Portions

Serve food on modest-sized plates – and don't skimp on the fruit and veggies!

5: Inspire Your Child to Enjoy Daily Physical Activity

Encourage your family to enjoy a minimum of 60 minutes of moderate-intensity physical activity per day.

6: Nurture a Wrap-around Family Lifestyle

Create a wrap-around home environment that supports healthy food and lifestyle choices. Eat family meals together as a regular practise. Practise healthy cooking and eating as an example for your children.

7: Be Your Child's Lifestyle Authority

Communicate food and lifestyle habits to your children in an authoritative rather than an authoritarian style.

PART 3

Japanese Inspirations for Family Meals

1

The Typical Japanese Meal

You can be healthy with foods inspired by any nation or culture, and I think that today we have a wide range of foods and tastes to explore, as people move to different countries, bringing with them their culinary cultures from around the world. In this chapter I briefly describe the basic concept of a typical Japanese meal structure. In the next chapter I will explain the key ingredients for Japanese cooking, and I hope you will be tempted to try some of them in the recipes that follow.

Let's first look at the culinary heritage that makes the cuisine of Japan so fascinating, along with its typical meal structure.

One soup and three dishes – a typical Japanese meal

Ichi-jyu san-sai is a typical Japanese meal structure, consisting of a bowl of soup, three side dishes (with varieties of vegetables and protein), a bowl of rice and a plate of fruit as a dessert. The vast majority of Japanese dishes are variations on five simple but highly versatile themes: fish, soya, rice, vegetables and fruit. Meat is popular in Japan, too, but in smaller portions and less frequently than in the West.

The classic Japanese home-cooked meal consists of a piece of grilled fish, a bowl of rice, simmered or vinegared vegetables, a serving of miso soup, sliced seasonal fruit for dessert and a cup of hot tea. In the most basic sense, a typical Japanese home-cooked meal means simply a bowl of rice, a bowl of soup, and three side dishes. These dishes are served at the same time, not as separate courses.

The idea is to eat little bites of each dish alternately. Parents (and in multigenerational households, grandparents) typically encourage the children to eat a little bit of everything and to chew every mouthful well to aid good digestion.

Breakfast

A typical Japan-style breakfast consists of foods such as cooked rice, miso soup with small cubes of tofu and spring onions, small sheets of nori sea vegetable, a small omelette or piece of grilled salmon, a side dish of vegetables, a side dish of fruit, with green tea to drink or water, non-caffeinated barley tea or milk for children.

A Japanese-style breakfast gives you a huge dose of sustained energy and nutrition to last the morning; in contrast to many high-calorie, high-sugar and low-nutrient Western breakfasts, which can lead to you feeling sleepy and hungry again.

Japanese people have adopted Western-style breakfast items, too. They may have toasted bread for breakfast with eggs, sausages or slices of ham and cheeses, although these will be in much smaller portions than in the West, plus coffee or black tea with lemon or milk (a glass of milk, water or unsweetened mugicha – barley tea – for children), a salad or sautéed vegetables, and fruit.

My mother in Tokyo, for example, also serves toasted bread for breakfast, but it is always accompanied with a healthy portion of vegetables such as a freshly made salad, and sautéed vegetables with a small amount of meat as a garnish and/or a sunny-side-up pan-fried egg. Alternatively, she will serve a large bowl of vegetable and egg soup plus fruit. The Japanese eat muffins, pastries, or sugary cereals for breakfast much less frequently than in the West. These are considered 'sweets' and for occasional treats only, enjoyed in small portions.

Lunch

The midday Japan-style meal can be something simple like a bowl of soba noodles with tempura, fish, or seasonal mountain vegetables, a bowl of rice topped with grilled meat and vegetables and a bowl of miso soup, or onigiri – rice balls and miso soup, with side dishes. Lunch boxes, called bento, are a portable version of the typical Japanese meal of rice and three side dishes packed in a lunchbox.

Dinner

The evening meal is often more elaborate, but it follows the same pattern: rice, soup and various side dishes of meat, fish, soya and vegetables.

A daily menu

Below is a sample daily menu to help you visualise the typical Japanese meal structure. I hope that it will help you to create Japanese-style menus of your own if you would like to try out some of the recipes in Chapter 4 of Part 3 for your family.

Breakfast

A bowl of haiga-mai rice
A bowl of miso soup with chunks of tofu, wakame sea
   vegetables and chopped spring onions
A small piece of grilled salmon
A small piece of omelette
A variety of simmered local, seasonal vegetables
A cup of water, green tea or mugicha (barley tea)

Lunch

A bowl of hot soba (buckwheat noodles) topped with usu-age (thin slices of fried tofu), gently boiled, crisp-tender spinach, and chopped spring onions and shredded nori sea vegetables as garnishes

A serving of edamame (soya beans)

A cup of water, green tea, or mugicha

Dinner

A bowl of brown rice

A bowl of miso soup with daikon (mooli), leafy greens and chopped spring onions

One-pot Beef, Potato and Onion Casserole (page 149)

Aubergines and Red Peppers with Sweet Red Miso Sauce (page 174)

Simmered tofu chunks served with Sweet Dashi–Soy Seasoning Sauce (page 184)

A cup of water, green tea or mugicha

2

Choosing the Healthiest Ingredients

When choosing ingredients, I recommend that whenever possible, you buy fresh, locally grown or produced organic produce in season. This way of sourcing food ingredients is one of the essential concepts of Japanese cuisine.

Really fresh ingredients provide maximum flavour. Their colours are vivid, the textures are crisp and firm, and the aromas are bursting and pleasing to all the senses.

Organically grown foods, of course, bring maximum purity, meaning a much lower level of chemical substances. Organic farming requires agricultural techniques that are more ecologically balanced.

Having said that, it's important to note that all forms of veggies and fruit are healthy – fresh, canned or frozen – provided there is a wide variety of different types eaten and they are prepared healthfully, and with minimal added salt and sugar.

The benefits of locally sourced, fresh, organic and seasonal foods

In recent years, more people have become aware of the importance of buying local food. It supports local farmers and businesses and it often reduces the costs of the produce, because overseas and long-distance transportation and storage expenses are eliminated. It is often kinder to the earth because it reduces the emissions of carbon dioxide and other greenhouse gases from fossil-fuel-based transport. And, best of all, it allows you to buy products that have been harvested as close as possible to their optimum ripeness. Often, when you shop at a market or your local greengrocer and go for seasonal produce, you are buying vegetables and fruits that were picked early that morning, and you could be eating some of them for dinner on the same day.

Produce in season can be cheaper than the same produce bought out of season and sourced from outside the country you live in, as it is available in abundance, and it will taste better as well. Serving seasonal foods brings variety – different flavours, colours, shapes and textures – to your family meals.

Particular foods can signal to you and your children the arrival of a new season. As your children grow up, some foods might trigger memories associated with certain activities related to different seasons. For me, every time I see a mountain of gigantic watermelons in a store, I remember summer scenes from my childhood. One is of many evenings after dinner, Papa, my little sister Miki and I sitting on a wooden veranda overlooking the backyard, enjoying the tiniest bit of cool breeze in the hot air, while Mum brought out a watermelon, a knife and a chopping board on a tray. She would cut up the melon and arrange the slices on the tray. We all enjoyed cool, sweet, juicy and fresh watermelon one bite after another – us kids spitting the seeds into the backyard.

Feasting on local, seasonal produce is a wonderful way to experience the essence of the season and to be in sync with the harmony of nature. One easy and exciting way to buy fresh, organic, local produce in season is to go to your local farmers' market, but you will also find it in street markets, local greengrocers and some wholefood shops that also stock fresh produce. Subscribing to a weekly green box is another way to be sure you are getting fresh, local produce. The choices will change from week to week, unlike the monotonous selections in supermarkets, where everything is available all year. Many small-scale growers who sell their produce at markets and local shops do not have the resources to apply for organic certification but they often practise sustainable agricultural techniques or grow without using chemicals. In this case, I prefer to buy locally grown vegetables rather than certified organic produce that has been harvested thousands of miles away.

Buying meat and fish

As for buying meat, poultry, dairy and eggs, I suggest that, as often as possible, you choose products derived from animals that have been pasture-fed, or fed organic feed, and treated humanely and without antibiotics.

When buying seafood, look for fresh, local fish and shellfish in season that has been sustainably caught wherever possible. For a complete UK guide on which kinds of fish to buy and which to avoid, check out the Marine Conservation Society website: http://www.fishonline.org/. And for other nations, go to the international resource list at: http://www.seafoodwatch.org/resources.

When buying fish for babies and children, the NHS does not recommend that children under 16 eat shark, swordfish or marlin because the levels of mercury in these fish can affect a child's nervous system. Raw shellfish is unsuitable for babies and children because of the risk of food poisoning.

For other fish, always remove the bones before serving it to children, and be particularly careful to remove bones when giving it to young children. Bones and skin in canned fish, like Alaskan salmon, however, are soft and edible, and are a good source of calcium.

Japanese storecupboard ingredients

Not all foods can be bought locally or in season. For those other items, stock your storecupboard and freezer with canned, jarred, frozen and dried products. They are economical and convenient, and they are also nutritious. Here are some examples of particular items we have in our storecupboard and freezer:

- Canned tomatoes, tomato purée and sun-dried tomato paste (for tomato-based sauces, soups and stews)
- Canned and frozen beans (for soups, main and side dishes)
- Frozen vegetables (for soups, main and side dishes)
- Frozen edamame (for snacks, salads, main and side dishes)
- Canned and frozen fish, such as wild Alaskan salmon, kippers, sardines and mackerel (for quick omega-3-rich snacks and meals)
- Frozen vegetables such as broccoli and spinach (for side dishes)
- Frozen fruit, such as berries, peaches and mangoes (for desserts)
- Dried sea vegetables – kombu, wakame, hijiki and nori (for making dashi cooking stock, soups, salads, garnish, and main and side dishes)
- Dried mushrooms (for making dashi cooking stock, and main and side dishes)
- Dried Japanese vegetables such as daikon (mooli) (for main and side dishes)
- Dried fruits such as raisins and dates (for salads and snacks)

Look for ingredients without added salt, or choose low-salt options, if you can.

You may have a local Japanese grocer where you can buy the more unusual ingredients listed, but today many are stocked by major supermarkets as well as small ethnic markets or grocers. You may be surprised by what you can find nearby. Otherwise, you can buy most of the ingredients online.

The key ingredients demystified

Eating healthy meals does not require learning to cook authentic Japanese dishes or using ingredients popular in Japan, but it can make eating more exciting. The Japanese way of eating is one that is natural for Japanese children, who are served smaller portions of everything adults eat. By trying some of the ingredients and configuring Japanese-style meals, you will be adding variety to your family's overall dining experiences, and I hope you and your family will find the process enjoyable. As a result, I hope that you will also attain a deeper understanding of the seven secrets we discussed in the earlier chapters, and you and your family will have the joy of eating delicious, healthy meals for many years to come.

Many Japanese ingredients are now becoming more commonplace, as Japanese-influenced cooking becomes mainstream, and so it is increasingly easy to locate ingredients such as yuzu, wasabi, miso and shiitake, which are grown and produced outside of Japan. In the UK, for example, NamaYasai Farm in East Sussex grows Japanese vegetables and sells them at their local farmers' market in Lewes, but they also have green box collection points in various parts of the south east. If you have a local ethnic market or supermarket, you may find many of the Japanese items there.

3

Discovering Japanese Ingredients

Most of the ingredients listed here are packaged, so they are storecupboard ingredients that you can use in a number of dishes.

Barley is a versatile, delicious, healthy and easy-to-cook grain option to be added to the pantry. It is a wonderful addition especially for families with children. It is versatile, as it mixes so well with practically any type of dish and cuisine. You can add it to rice – not only premium Japanese short-grain rice but also other varieties like basmati, sprouted tricolour blend and wild rice. Use these mixed grains in leafy green and sea vegetable salads, Japanese and Western soups, and for onigiri rice balls. Mix it into Japanese premium short-grain rice and use it in hamburgers, dumplings and sushi-rolls. Its flavour is subtle and its texture is slightly chewy, like al dente pasta, giving a delightful layer to a grain mix and adding volume to dishes like salads and soups.

Barley is a champion of good nutrition. It is jam-packed with fibre (2.8 times more compared to brown rice, and 17 times compared to white rice), it contains vital vitamins and minerals and is low in fat. Like other whole grains, it can help you lose weight as part of a healthy diet, assist digestive health and reduce the risk of cardiovascular diseases.

Bonito (fish) flakes (katsuobushi, hana-katsuo or kezuribushi)
A member of the mackerel family, bonito generally makes its appearance in Japanese cuisine not as a whole fish but as dried bonito fish flakes. These fish flakes, or katsuobushi, are an important ingredient in the Japanese kitchen. The larger fish flakes are used to make dashi, the essential cooking stock (page 181), while the smaller flakes are used as a garnish for many dishes. Bonito flakes look like paper-thin curls of wood and range in colour from pinky-beige to dark burgundy.

Although some Japanese people make their own fish flakes with a special bonito-shaving implement, you can buy commercially shaved flakes in clear plastic bags. Large flakes for making dashi range in quantities from 28g (1oz) to 450g (1lb) bags. The small fish flakes typically used for garnishes come in single-serving packets, usually five to a bag, with individual packets weighing from 15g (½oz) to 28g (1oz). Bonito flakes have a mild, smoky, faintly sweet flavour. Although it's probably unlike anything you've encountered in Western cooking, it's a taste that's easy to acquire.

Daikon (mooli or white radish) is a large, white Japanese radish. It is quite juicy and has a fresh, sweet flavour and a mild bite. It is one of my favourite vegetables in winter. It is so versatile, it can be used in salads, simmered dishes, and pickled and grated to use as a garnish. Raw grated daikon is usually served as a garnish with oily foods because the moist radish provides an ideal counterpoint to deep-fried foods such as tempura and fatty fish, much the way that lemon does in Western cooking. Gently simmered chunky daikon served with sweetened miso paste is delicious. Daikon also makes a tasty addition to miso soup – turning soft and almost sweet as it simmers in the savoury liquid. Some daikon can be spicy (mild to hot) when it is raw – you may want to taste it before you serve it to young children.

When buying for freshness, look out for the fresh, green spiky leaves with the ends of the roots intact. Choose daikon that are firm, not limp. I love to eat the stem-leaf portion as much as the root. The stems are crunchy and the leaves are peppery. They taste wonderful in stir-fries with other vegetables and miso soup. You can substitute salad radishes if you are unable to locate daikon.

Edamame (fresh green soya beans) have become a popular appetiser at restaurants and parties in the West. The fresh beans are available during the summer months at selected shops and farmers' markets. If you can't find fresh edamame, the frozen ones, in their pods or without, make a fine, convenient substitute. They make a fantastic instant snack and side dish for children.

Hon-mirin (the genuine mirin, to differentiate it from artificially produced seasoning products sold with mirin-style flavour claims) is a sweet, golden cooking wine, made from glutinous rice, and it has an alcohol content of about 14 per cent. The alcohol is burned off during cooking, so it's safe to use in meals for children. It is bought in a bottle and is used in many Japanese home-style recipes. Hon-mirin has several benefits. It adds sweetness, deep, full-bodied umami to simmered dishes and sauces. Its sweetness is subtle compared to that of sugar, bringing a classy, delicate sweetness to dishes. Hon-mirin makes luscious glazes, for example, a perfect finishing touch to fillets of white fish. It also prevents chunks of foods like potatoes and fish from breaking into pieces while being simmered, and it helps the flavours penetrate into foods.

Japanese sweet potato (also called bushbok, white flesh sweet potato, kumara, Asian sweet potato) has historically been very popular in Japan. It has pinkish-purple skin with white flesh. It is one of the tastiest and most nutritious members of the pantheon of vegetables. It is nutty tasting like chestnuts, unlike Western sweet potatoes with orange flesh. It is extremely nutritious, packed with potassium, vitamin C and dietary fibre. My seven-year-old son eats it as one of his almost-daily snacks and/or as a side dish. He loves to eat sweet potato cut into stick shapes and baked (pages 178 and 179) – no dips or sauces required. It's far and away his favourite vegetable. I serve them almost every time he has a playdate, and so far every child has asked for more. If cooked properly, it has a scrumptious taste that any child would enjoy. When buying, look for firm sweet potatoes with smooth skins and no soft spots. Don't put them in a plastic bag, or in the fridge; store them in a dry, cool and dark place. All sweet potatoes are nutritional superstars, not just the Japanese kind, and can be used in any of the following recipes where Japanese sweet potatoes are specified.

Miso is a thick, salty fermented soya-bean paste that looks something like peanut butter and is bought in pouches or plastic tubs. It is made from crushed soya beans, salt, a fermenting agent and the addition of barley, rice or wheat. Depending on which grain is added, the miso will vary tremendously in flavour, texture, aroma and colour. Miso can range in flavour from salty to sweet, in texture from smooth to slightly pebbly or chunky (with the addition of crushed grains or soya beans), in smell from delicate to pungent, and in colour from beige to golden yellow to brown.

In its many variations, miso is a staple of the Japanese kitchen and adds a savoury base note to soups, dressings, simmered dishes and stir-fries. White miso is actually a pale yellow and has a milder, sweeter flavour than other miso varieties. Because of its delicate nature, it's often used for dressings (particularly for vegetables) and in marinades for mild-tasting fish and seafood. Red miso, which is rusty brown in colour, is coarser and saltier than white. It works best in marinades and sauces for meats. The darkest brown version of red miso has the sharpest flavour and tastes best when added to simmered dishes containing oily fish or hearty meats. There are also mixed red-and-white versions of miso.

For miso soup as well as other dishes, many Japanese cooks keep two or three different kinds of miso in the fridge so that they can combine them to achieve their preferred taste. Restaurant chefs around the world have discovered the magic of miso and are using it to add a savoury flavour to boost a variety of dishes – not just Asian ones. Like soy sauce, miso can sometimes be very high in salt, so look for lower-salt or reduced-salt miso by carefully reading the label. Store miso in an airtight container in the fridge once opened.

Mitsuba, also known as trefoil or Japanese parsley, is a pretty garnish. I have included it in several of the recipes in this book, although flat-leaf parsley is fine to use in its place.

Nira is a member of the chive family and is also known as Chinese chives or garlic chives. The green leaves are flat, unlike the round chives commonly sold in the UK. I like their bold flavour – stronger than that of onions, but subtler than garlic. Substitute nira with shallots or chives. Nira also makes a great ingredient for stir-fry dishes.

Noodles Japan is awash with noodles. Japanese noodles fall into two major camps: those made with buckwheat flour (soba) and those made with white wheat flour (udon). Children love noodles just as they do pasta! Egg noodles, or **ramen**, originally Chinese, are also very popular in Japan, mostly enjoyed as packet instant soups, in specialist ramen shops, many of which have become a craze in big cities such as New York and London in recent years.

Soba is the name for noodles made from buckwheat flour. Soba is a Japanese nutrition champion – a good source of protein, whole grains, fibre and complex carbohydrates. The noodles are thin, greyish brown and delightfully nutty tasting with a silky smooth texture. They are served hot in soups, as well as cold with a tasty sweet soya dipping sauce. Because buckwheat flour lacks gluten, the component in wheat flour that gives noodles their pleasant chewiness, most noodle makers add a little bit of starch to the dough. Some soba manufacturers add too much starch (in the form of white wheat flour or yam flour) – mainly to cut costs, because buckwheat flour costs more than other flours. The result is an inferior soba noodle that lacks the distinctive earthy flavour. Look for noodles that are as close to 100 per cent buckwheat as possible, or at least 80 per cent buckwheat and 20 per cent wheat. Clearspring is a brand worth looking for. Among soba purists, these dark brown noodles are considered the best.

One of the most popular kinds of white flour noodle, especially among children, is **udon**. They are thick and white and have a wonderful chewy texture. Udon are eaten hot in soups with a variety of toppings, or cold with dipping sauce. One thing to be careful of when buying dry or frozen udon noodles at grocery stores is to choose low-salt or 'no salt added' ones. Surprisingly, the majority of udon products contain too much salt. Because they are served with a soya sauce-based broth, which is salty, it's important not to use salted noodles. Look out for a brand like Hakubaku, which sells salt-free and organic noodles. Other tasty white flour noodles you might see in a Japanese store include **kishimen**, which are chewy, flat and wide, almost like fettuccine.

Somen are a snow-white noodle as thin as angel-hair pasta and almost always served cold in the summer. A slightly thicker version of somen is **hiyamugi**.

I think fresh noodles taste the best. Throughout Japan, trained noodle masters sell hand-made soba and udon from their shops. In major cities like New York, London, Sydney and Melbourne, there are superb, handmade Japanese noodles at premium noodle speciality restaurants. I highly recommend trying hand made soba, if you can, to expand your culinary horizon. In the UK, a Japanese female master Manami Koshiba at Sobauchi London offers soba-making lessons (students must be at least 11 years old as a class uses an oversized knife). Because it's hard to find fresh soba and udon at grocery stores in the West, all the noodle recipes in this book call for dried noodles. High-quality dried soba and udon are readily available and very tasty. The recipes in this book use only soba and udon noodles.

Oils Polyunsaturates, and to a lesser extent, monounsaturates, have been shown to lower blood cholesterol levels and therefore help in reducing the risk of heart disease. It is better to eat foods rich in monounsaturates (olive oil and rapeseed oil) and polyun-saturates (sunflower oil and soya oil), than foods rich in saturates. The Japanese mostly use vegetable oils to cook. Leading varieties are rapeseed (called canola in Japan) and soya, and others include corn, cotton, safflower, rice bran, sunflower, sesame and olive.

Rapeseed oil contains mostly monounsaturated fat and is a good and cheaper alternative to olive oil. It is one of the best vegetable oils to cook with, because it has among the highest concentrations of polyunsaturated fat and monounsaturated fat and a low level of saturated fat. Except in its hydrogenated form, it has absolutely none of the worst fat of all: trans-fat. Because rapeseed oil has little flavour, due to its processing method, it allows the pure natural flavour of ingredients to shine through, which is one of the core principles of Japanese cooking. The combined health benefit and absence of strong flavour makes rapeseed oil the leading cooking oil choice in Japan. Look for non-hydrogenated rapeseed oil.

Extracted from sesame seeds, **sesame oil** comes in two types: light and dark (also called toasted). The lighter oil has a softer flavour and colour than the dark version. Its potent flavour makes it appropriate to use as a garnish. Sesame oil can be used as a cooking oil. Tempura recipes often call for half sesame oil and half vegetable oil. I love to sprinkle it on stir-fried vegetables as soon as I turn off the heat and I also use it in my salad dressings for its nutty flavour and aroma.

Panko, Japanese breadcrumbs, is a modern ingredient which makes a light, crunchy crust. (The term is a fusion of the French word for bread, *pain*, with *ko*, which means 'powder' in Japanese.) Unlike the breadcrumbs you are probably used to, panko has a texture that is more like flakes than crumbs. Typical home-cooked dishes that are very popular among children are potato croquettes and tonkatsu: breaded pork cutlets, although panko is not used in the recipes in this book.

Rice Short-grain white rice is used as standard for Japanese home cooking. It is moister and stickier than medium and long-grain rice. Short-grain brown rice, or genmai, is a wholegrain, high-fibre alternative. A third option, haiga-mai (literally, rice-germ rice), is partially polished to remove only its bran, the tough fibrous outer layer, and keep the germ, the most nutritious portion of the grain, intact (this part is usually removed in the milling process for white rice). For families with children, unless you are already eating brown rice, I recommend haiga-mai as the optimum option, and gradually introduce brown rice as the children grow (not before five years of age) and are accustomed to a more wholegrain-based diet. I find haiga-mai tastes more nutty than polished white rice, but not quite as hearty as brown. Unlike the other rice types, haiga-mai should *not* be rinsed before cooking, in order to preserve the germ.

Premium varieties of short-grain rice popular among Japanese are koshihikari, hitomebore and akita-komachi. The champion variety, koshihikari, is traditionally grown in Japan and sold under a number of different brand labels. It will be a delightful addition to your meals for its superior flavour and texture. Koshi-hikari is now cultivated in the US, Australia and New Zealand, and it is available in the UK. I have found that these rices are just as tasty as Japanese-grown rice. It is certainly less expensive and more sustainable than buying rice imported from Japan. You might occasionally want to splurge on the award-winning Uonumasan Koshihikari brand, grown in the region of Uonuma, Niigata, Japan, or try other premium varieties.

Store all rice in an airtight container in a cool, dry place, for up to a year.

Rice vinegar In addition to the fried, steamed and simmered categories of Japanese cooking, there is a fourth category: vinegared dishes, typically served as starters or side dishes. The rice vinegar used in these dishes is made either from white rice or brown rice. Regular rice vinegar ranges in colour from light to golden yellow, whereas brown rice vinegar ranges from brown to black.

Brown rice vinegar tastes milder than regular rice vinegar – yet rice vinegar overall has much less of a bite than pungent Western vinegars. Even when I'm making Western-style salads, I prefer to make my dressings with rice vinegar, since it's not as sour as white or red wine vinegar. If you have ever eaten sushi, you are already familiar with the taste of rice vinegar, since the sushi rice is gently tossed with a mixture of rice vinegar, sugar and salt.

Rice wine is also called sake, and is made from fermented rice grains. It not only makes a delightful alcoholic drink but it also adds an indispensable touch to many Japanese dishes. Sake adds depth to simmered dishes, sauces and dressings and it reduces fish and meat odours. Sake is available in numerous styles and it ranges enormously in quality, price and flavour, from dry to quite sweet. Since the alcohol in sake evaporates during cooking, you can still cook with it even if you avoid alcohol, and you can use it for dishes for children; however, I do not use sake in the recipes in this book.

Sea vegetables – seaweed – are nutritious, tasty and extremely versatile, and they play an integral role in the Japanese diet. They are rich in iodine, folate, magnesium, iron, calcium, riboflavin and pantothenic acid. Sea-vegetable flavoured stocks are found in cold salads and add a savoury crunch to rice and noodle dishes. **Kombu**, also known as konbu or kobu, is considered the king of seaweeds in Japan. A kind of kelp, it is thick, leafy and brownish green. Outside of Japan, kombu is primarily available dried, often in rectangles ranging in size from 2.5 × 13cm (1 × 5in) to 13 × 25cm (5 × 10in) for use in the clear cooking stock dashi where it is steeped in water with dried bonito flakes. Dashi stock (page 182) is used as the base for many Japanese dishes. Kombu is also enjoyed simmered (as an accompaniment to white rice) and dried as a snack.

    Nori refers to the thin, flat sheets of dried seaweed that range in colour from pine green to purple-black. If you've ever eaten sushi rolls, you've tasted nori. It's the crackly dark green substance that wraps around the vinegared rice (and eventually becomes soft and slightly chewy the longer it sits).

A popular Japanese snack that uses nori is onigiri, or rice balls (page 161). Every convenience store in Japan has a section devoted to these small vegetable- or fish-stuffed rice balls (or triangles) sealed with nori. Nori, used to make sushi, is often toasted and is bought labelled 'sushi nori'. Toasting enhances the flavour and crisp texture of the seaweed. Sushi nori is usually bought in 20cm (8in) squares with several sheets to a bag. Because nori loses its crispness as soon as it is exposed to the air, remove only one sheet at a time for whatever you're making and keep the bag sealed at all times. To store, put the nori in an airtight container or zip-lock bag.

Shredded nori makes a popular garnish for rice and noodle dishes. You can buy containers of commercially cut nori, or make your own, cutting a sheet of nori into a pile of 5mm × 2.5cm (¼ × 1in) strips (or squares, as I sometimes do). Seasoned nori sheets are also available. The crisp sheets are brushed with a sweet soy-based sauce and often sold in small rectangles with only a few sheets to each packet. Seasoned nori sheets wrapped around hot cooked rice are a popular Japanese breakfast treat and are easy to make. You simply take a small sheet of seasoned nori and quickly dip one side in some soy sauce. Then, wrap the seaweed around a mouthful of rice from your rice bowl. Alternatively, tear the seasoned nori into small bits and scatter them over your rice.

Wakame is a common sea vegetable in Japan. It is used in soups, salads and toppings for soba noodles. When you have miso soup at a Japanese restaurant, the chances are that it comes with a few ribbons of wakame. In Japan, you can buy fresh wakame as long green leaves. Outside Japan, you can buy the dried version – dark green strands in a plastic bag.

Sesame seeds In Japanese home cooking, white and black sesame seeds (goma) add a fragrant, nutty accent to all kinds of dishes. I recommend buying whole untoasted sesame seeds. The seeds are used to garnish vegetable, tofu, seafood and meat dishes, as well as to flavour dipping sauces. Grinding the seeds turns them into a flaky base used for dressings and sauces. Most Japanese cooks grind their sesame seeds with a wooden pestle in a ribbed ceramic bowl called a *suribachi*. You can grind them in a food processor, or with a pestle and mortar. Or you can buy sesame seeds already ground.

Shichimi togarashi is a mixture of seven spices, which adds a spicy, peppery flavour to foods. It is a distinctly Japanese blend of ground red pepper, roasted orange peel, white and black sesame seeds, sanshō, seaweed and ginger. You could use cayenne or chilli powder, if you cannot find shichimi togarashi, but it will simply add a kick of heat to dishes versus the burst of heat and flavour you get from the combination of the seven spices. You will find that occasionally I suggest serving a dish with shichimi togarashi for the adults.

Shiso is a herb from the mint family. Shiso leaves are quite fragrant with a slightly bitter, mint-like flavour and measure about 5cm (2in) square. Heart-shaped with jagged edges, shiso grows in green and reddish-purple varieties. Whole shiso leaves are commonly used in Japan as a garnish for sashimi and as an ingredient in tempura. Finely chopped leaves are used as a seasoning for tofu and other dishes, and the dried chopped red leaves can be sprinkled on hot rice for flavouring. In early summer, pale pink shiso flowers on a short stem are used as a decorative and edible seasonal garnish. All shiso leaves used in my recipes are the green and fresh kind.

Soy sauce, or shoyu, is a Japanese home-style cooking workhorse. This dark-brown liquid, derived from soya beans, barley (or wheat), salt and water, has a distinctive savoury richness that gives Japanese cooking its signature flavour. In addition to seasoning soups, sauces, marinades and dressings, soy sauce serves as an indispensable condiment for dishes such as sushi;

however, soy sauce should be used with a delicate hand. Many Westerners make the mistake of saturating their food with it, not realising that a little goes a very long way. When used properly and sparingly, soy sauce should bring out, not overwhelm, the innate flavour of an ingredient.

I suggest you use reduced-salt (or light) soy sauce. To me, reduced-salt soy sauce tastes just as good as, if not better than, regular soy sauce. Many supermarkets carry reduced-salt soy sauce, and all the recipes in this book call for reduced-salt soy sauce. A high-quality wheat-free alternative to soy sauce that's popular among health-food devotees and people with wheat allergies is tamari. It tastes similar to soy sauce and also comes in reduced-salt varieties.

Tea Caffeine-free mugicha is **barley tea**, which is a great substitute for the sweetened and carbonated beverages that Westerners favour. It has a smooth, mild and subtly sweet flavour, making it the champion of daily beverages for children. Most of the Japanese mothers I spoke to for this book serve water and/or cold unsweetened mugicha to their children to quench their thirst. When made cold, it is a healthy and refreshing summertime drink.

Tofu is coagulated soya milk, made from soya beans and cut into blocks. Most tofu is white with a hint of light yellow, like vanilla ice cream. Tofu is extremely popular in Japan. It's a sort of meat-and-potatoes ingredient for most Japanese home cooks, and there are hundreds of delicious ways to prepare it. Among tofu's many merits is its high protein content. As a result, it makes a terrific substitute for all kinds of meat, poultry and seafood. When it's of good quality, it has a subtle, clean and lightly earthy taste.

I believe that tofu is one of the most children-friendly Japanese food items: it's soft and easy to eat, even for babies who are starting solids, and you can add a flavour that your child likes because tofu has very little taste of its own.

Tofu is incredibly versatile. It can be added to starters, soups, main courses, dressings, sauces and desserts, and it can be eaten on its own – hot or cold – with various garnishes. Tofu also has a wide variety of textures, depending upon how it has been prepared. Steaming, for example, turns tofu plump and juicy, whereas stir-frying turns it crispy, firm and golden. When stewed, tofu becomes tender and succulent, and when whipped in a blender or food processor, it becomes creamy and thick, like soured cream.

When you want to add another dish to your menu, look for a simple tofu recipe. It is a delicious, filling, healthy protein booster. Keep a block of tofu in the fridge, or a tetra-pack in a cupboard.

Tofu is sold in various forms. The two basic kinds are known as 'silken' and 'cotton', and both may come in different degrees of firmness. Since the language used by different manufacturers to describe the several variations within those two general categories is not always consistent, here are some general directions to help you navigate through the tofu landscape.

Silken tofu, or kinugoshi tofu, is extremely delicate, with a porcelain-like colour and a custard-pudding-like texture both outside and inside. This lovely texture is achieved because silken tofu, unlike the cotton types, is coagulated without being pressed to eliminate excess water. Silken tofu is used in elegant soups or chilled and eaten on its own with various garnishes. Because silken tofu is so delicate, it needs careful handling. A traditional way is to take the fragile tofu block directly from the container and to slip it onto the palm of your hand, then use the other hand to cut the tofu very carefully with a knife into smaller pieces. You can then slide the tofu with great care onto a plate or into water or broth that is gently simmering in a saucepan. All of this gentle handling is for the purpose of making sure that the tofu remains intact in little squares, which look pretty floating, for example, in a clear soup. You would find that if you cut the silken tofu on a chopping board, some pieces might break up when they are transferred from the chopping board to the saucepan or the plate.

Silken tofu is sold in airtight plastic containers with water, or in aseptic packaging without water. The waterless packaging means that it can keep indefinitely on the shelf. The water-packed variety has a shorter shelf life and should be used as soon as it is opened.

Cotton (as it's known in Japan) or firm tofu is less fragile than silken and, the 'firm' designation notwithstanding, it comes in textures generally labelled soft, medium-firm, firm and extra-firm. Generally speaking, the recipes in this book that call for cotton tofu use the firm texture, although that is more a matter of taste than necessity.

The process of making cotton tofu involves separating the curds from the whey of the soya milk and then compressing the curds. This is what makes the texture of cotton tofu so much firmer (even in its so-called soft versions). Cotton tofu has a slightly coarse surface and a much more substantial bite and texture than silken, which makes it suitable for stir-fries and for grilled and simmered dishes (page 151).

Thick, fried tofu rectangles (about 7 × 12 × 2.5cm/2¾ × 4½ × 1in) are known as astu-age tofu. Thin, fried tofu rectangles (about 7 × 12 × 0.5cm/4 × 4½ × ¼in) are known as atsu-age tofu. Both thin and thick fried tofu are golden yellow on the outside. My son loves usu-age tofu in inari sushi and kitsune udon (pages 167 and 171).

Yakidofu tofu is firm cotton tofu that has been grilled and has scorch marks on the surface. It is packed in water in a plastic container, and it tastes a little smoky. It is used in sukiyaki dishes in Japan.

Because all tofu is quite perishable, be sure to use it within a few days of opening the package. Once opened, store it in the fridge submerged in cold water in a covered container.

Wasabi is a well-known Japanese condiment in the UK. It suffuses the palate with a mixture of spice and heat. Unlike horseradish, which grows in soil, wasabi grows in cold, shallow streams high in the mountains of Japan. The rhizome portion of the wasabi plant, which is the edible part, is about 2.5cm (1in) in diameter and ranges from 8cm to 15cm (3in to 6in) long. Wasabi is expensive to harvest and cultivate, which is why most shops sell a cheap substitute under the wasabi name. If you've ever eaten sushi or sashimi at a modestly priced Japanese restaurant, the chances are you've been served a small cone of light green paste fabricated primarily from mustard and/or horseradish powder and green food colouring. It's acrid, fiery and flavourless and bears little resemblance to freshly grated wasabi. Fresh wasabi is now harvested outside of Japan. Look for local growers and add it to your special-occasion meals. In the UK, you can order it online from The Wasabi Company in Dorset, who supply their fresh wasabi to top-tier restaurant chefs.

Beyond its use in sushi and sashimi, wasabi often accompanies cold soba noodles, chilled tofu and various fish and grilled chicken dishes. You might have also seen wasabi-flavoured peas and nori sold as snack items in supermarkets. Although not suitable for children, I have suggested serving some of the dishes with wasabi for the adults.

Yuzu is a popular citrus fruit. Its rind and juice are used to add a citrus aroma and sour taste to numerous Japanese dishes. Bottled yuzu juice is sold at specialist Japanese shops. Fresh lime or lemon makes a good substitute.

4

Japanese-style Recipes for Families

I hope that you will feel inspired by this book to try some of these Japan-inspired family-and-child-friendly recipes. The flavours may be different from the ones your child may be familiar with, but I have included recipes that are some of my favourites from when I was growing up in Japan; recipes that I think you and your family may love. Just like a mother's Sunday roast, a father's BBQ, or a grandmother's Italian sauce in different parts of the world, recipes of traditional Japanese home-made dishes reflect different regional characteristics. They are handed down from generation to generation, and home cooks might incorporate recipes from other sources, such as their friends and relatives, or from cooking shows, magazines and websites.

The recipes are either my mother's or my own, and are often based on staple dishes of Japanese home cooking. Since my mother does not refer to written recipes (because they are all in her head) and she often improvises, hers were re-created, tested and written up based on her notes, comments and explanations. I modified them to accommodate my preferences for ingredients and dietary patterns; for example, they call for low-salt and/or no-added-salt products, and use less salt, soya sauces, miso and sugar – and less animal fats.

Sometimes I have suggested a little more seasoning to be added at the table for the adults or older children.

As for Western recipes such as biscuits and muffins, proportions have been tweaked and many substitutions have been applied; for example, oil for butter; wholegrain flours for white flour; soya, buckwheat, quinoa and/or coconut flours for wheat flours; and fruit, honey and/or agave nectar for sugar. A small amount of flaxseeds/chia seeds and vegetable purées are added to almost all of my baked goods and pancakes.

I encourage you to do the same. Take your family recipes, and change the proportions and make substitutions in favour of veggies, fruit and whole grains. If you're making pasta for dinner, try wholewheat, or quinoa pasta for the family if you have children of five years and older. Increase both the number and quantity of vegetables in a sauce and use less meat. Go light on salt. Serve the pasta on a medium-sized plate. Accompany it with a vegetable or pulse side dish and a clear soup with lots of vegetables and tofu and some meat as a garnish and to give flavour.

I hope you'll have fun involving your children in the shopping and preparation in your kitchen as well, and have a wrap-around lifestyle inspired by healthy food choices.

As we say in Japanese, *dozo, meshiagare* – enjoy!

Serving sizes

The recipes serve from **two to six adults**, as indicated. Assuming healthy choices like these, portion sizes for children should be guided by the parent's judgement. Leftovers can be covered and stored in the fridge for a healthy meal or snack.

A note on conversions

Metric and imperial measurements are given in the following recipes. The two are not exact conversions, however, so please follow one or the other but do not mix the two in the same recipe.

Soups

Miso Soup with Mussels

Shellfish with miso soup is a staple of home-cooked meals in Japan. The shells sticking out above the broth are such teases and invite diners to grab hold of their edges, ever so carefully so as not to burn their fingertips, or skilfully lift them up with chopsticks or a spoon. The aroma and steam rising from the broth has the ocean and earthy miso tones mingled in one, making the soup all the more appetising for the diners. I remember fondly asari, littleneck clams and shijimi, Asian clams often used in both miso and clear soups, and their distinct flavours emerging from my mother's Tokyo kitchen. I chose to use mussels for this recipe as they are not only delicious, but affordable, sustainable and locally available in the UK, Australia, New Zealand, Canada and many other parts of the world.

One of the fun things for children about eating shellfish is the process of separating the flesh from the shell. And this gives you incidental pauses in between bites and slows you down, helping you to eat mindfully. Serves 2

> 6 mussels in their shells
> 1 tbsp reduced-salt red or white miso
> 2 sprigs of mitsuba or flat-leaved parsley, knotted

1   Discard any mussels that do not close when sharply tapped. Scrub the mussels under cold water to remove any dirt from the shells, then rinse the mussels in several changes of water, until the water runs clear. To get rid of any grit inside the shells, soak the mussels in clean, cold water for 20 minutes. Remove the beard – the coarse threads protruding from the shells – by pulling it at the hinge, and discard it. Drain and rinse.

2   Put 750ml (26fl oz) cold water in a medium saucepan. Add the mussels. Bring the liquid to the boil. Skim the foam from the surface of the liquid using a ladle. The mussels are cooked as soon as they open, which should be only a few minutes after the water has come to the boil. Gently whisk in the miso until dissolved, then turn off the heat.

3   Discard any mussels that remain shut. Divide the mussels between two soup bowls. Ladle the soup over the mussels and garnish it with a knotted mitsuba sprig. Put a medium-sized bowl in the centre of the table for the discarded shells.

Miso Soup with Tofu and Spring Onions

Miso soup with small tofu cubes and chopped spring onions may be the typical miso soup variety around the world. If you've eaten at a casual Japanese restaurant and ordered a miso soup, most likely you will have found little chunks of tofu and spring onions in it. This recipe comes with a double-protein punch of miso and tofu, both made of soya beans. Tofu is one of the simplest food ingredients you can incorporate into your diet to provide Japanese-style eating for children. It's soft. It has virtually no flavour but it absorbs that of the broth. I recommend that you try tofu with the different kinds of firmness and find which kinds your family prefers. You can add chopped vegetables to make this soup more hearty and to boost your family's vegetable intake. Serves 2

700ml (1¼ pints) Dashi Stock (page 182)
1 spring onion, thinly sliced
125g (4½oz) firm tofu, rinsed and cut into small dice
1 tbsp reduced-salt red or white miso, or a combination of both

1   Put the dashi stock in a medium saucepan and bring to the boil. Stir in the spring onion and tofu, then bring the mixture back to the boil. Reduce the heat to medium and cook for 2 minutes or until the onion is tender. Gently whisk in the miso and turn off the heat. Ladle the soup into small bowls.

Miso Soup with Wakame

This is a good way to introduce the nutritious sea vegetable wakame into you child's diet. Serves 2

2 tbsp dried wakame
750ml (26fl oz) Dashi Stock (page 182)
1 spring onion, thinly sliced
1 tbsp reduced-salt red or white miso, or use a combination
of both

1   Soak the wakame in a medium bowl in 450ml (16fl oz) water for 15 minutes or until expanded and tender. Drain and cut into 3cm (1¼in) ribbons.

2   Put the dashi stock in a medium saucepan and bring to the boil. Stir in the wakame and spring onion, and bring the mixture back to the boil. Reduce the heat to medium and cook for 2 minutes or until the onion is tender.

3   Gently whisk in the miso and turn off the heat. Ladle the soup into two small soup bowls.

Japanese Sweet Potato, Pumpkin, Bean and Tomato Soup

This hearty stew–soup can be served as a stand-alone meal. It is naturally sweet, thanks to all the sweet vegetables in it. Since the vegetables are chopped small, children will enjoy many different flavours and textures in each mouthful. Serves 4

100g/4oz pearl barley
2 tbsp rapeseed, grapeseed or extra virgin olive oil
1 onion, chopped
1 carrot, chopped
1 celery stick, chopped
2 garlic cloves, crushed
180g (6¼oz) Japanese sweet potato (bushbok, white flesh, kumara, or regular sweet potato), peeled and cut into 1cm (½in) cubes

180g (6¼oz) kabocha squash or butternut squash, peeled and
cut into 1cm (½in) cubes with skin
1 litre (1¾ pints) Dashi Stock (page 182)
2 × 400g (14oz) cans chopped tomatoes, or 800g (1lb 12oz)
tomatoes, chopped
175g (6oz) tomato purée
400g (14oz) can cannellini beans, rinsed and drained
1 large handful fresh flat-leafed parsley, leaves chopped
4 tbsp chopped fresh basil

1　Cook the barley in a pan of boiling water for 30 minutes, or
according to the package instructions, until tender. Drain and
set aside. Preheat the oven to 180°C/350°F/Gas 4. Heat the oil
in a large flameproof casserole or ovenproof frying pan over
a medium heat. Add the onion, carrot, celery and garlic, and
cook for 5–7 minutes until the onions and celery are translucent to light brown.

2　Add the sweet potato and squash, and cook for 2 minutes more.
Add the dashi stock, tomatoes, tomato purée and beans, and
bring to the boil. Cover and put in the oven for 30 minutes or
until the vegetables are tender. Stir in the cooked barley. Stir in
the parsley and basil, and simmer for 2 minutes, before serving.

Sandwiches and Pizza

Sweet Avocado and Corn Sandwich

Ripe avocados are a nutrient-dense, convenient food for children
and a great source of 'good fat'. This avocado and corn sandwich
is an example of a simple but nutritious dish you can make for
your child. Serves 4

½ ripe avocado, pitted and flesh scooped out
1 tbsp ready-made apple sauce
2 tbsp canned cream-style sweetcorn
8 slices of wholemeal or white bread

1   Put the avocado in a small bowl and add the apple sauce and sweetcorn. Mash them together well. Divide the mixture into quarters. Spread each quarter of the mixture over 4 slices of the bread, then top with the remaining slices.

2   Neatly stack the 4 sandwiches on top of one another so that they are aligned, and gently press them down with the palm of your hand. If your child prefers the crusts cut off, do this now. If not, leave them on. Slice them into 4 long, stick shapes, for toddlers and young children, or triangles/rectangles for older children and adults.

Mini Pitta Pizza

A perfect way to serve more vegetables to a child, these pizzas make a delicious lunch or snack. And they are so easy to make. Makes 6

6 mini wholemeal pitta breads
6 tbsp All-purpose Vegetable Tomato Sauce (page 188)
6 tbsp grated mozzarella cheese
extra virgin olive oil, to drizzle

1   Preheat the oven to 220°C/425°F/Gas 7. Lay out the pitta breads on a baking sheet. Spread 1 tbsp of the tomato sauce onto each pitta bread using the back of a spoon. Sprinkle 1 tbsp of the cheese over each, then bake for 5–7 minutes until the cheese has melted. Drizzle some oil over each pizza. Serve whole, or cut into slices.

VARIATIONS Add different toppings. Try finely sliced onion, mushrooms, celery or olives; grated carrot or courgette; chopped baby spinach leaves, baby kale leaves, baby rocket leaves; small chunks of pineapple; sweetcorn, roasted peppers or beetroot; cooked seafood, slices of cooked chicken or turkey; chopped shiso, parsley or basil; toasted and ground sesame seeds or flaxseeds.

Salads

Chilled Cucumber Salad with Tofu and Chickpea Sauce

Serve this cooling salad for lunch or dinner during hot weather. The cucumbers are crisp-tender served with a delicious, mildly flavoured vegetable-protein sauce. Serves 2–4

200g (7oz) cucumber
a pinch of sea salt
50g (1¾oz) chilled Creamy Tofu and Chickpea Dipping Sauce (page 185)

1   Halve the cucumber and scoop out the seeds. Rub the salt onto the cucumber skin, then cut the cucumber diagonally into 5mm (¼in) slices. Put the cucumber into a colander, and leave it for 30 minutes for the salt to draw out the liquid, then squeeze out the remaining liquid.

2   Put the cucumber in a small bowl, add the tofu sauce and mix well. Serve immediately.

Summer Tomato and Tofu Salad

At the height of the summer, grab some ripe, sweet and juicy tomatoes at your local greengrocer, market or farmers' market. Look out for heritage tomatoes especially. These old varieties are exceptionally tasty. They are so full of flavour that you hardly need any dressings or condiments to serve with them. This recipe calls for vinaigrette, but that is to season the tofu. It's an amazing summer salad, which could become one of your child's summer-time favourites. Serves 2–4

200g (7oz) extra-firm tofu, rinsed and cut into 1cm (½in) cubes
2 ripe tomatoes, preferably heritage in different colours
1 tsp chopped fresh basil, shiso or flat-leaf parsley leaves

50ml (2fl oz) Traditional Japanese Sweet Vinegar Dressing
(page 185)
freshly ground black pepper (optional, for the adults)

1 Put the tofu cubes in a colander to drain off the excess water,
   cover and keep in the fridge until ready to use.

2 Cut out the cores of the tomatoes and cut the flesh into
   chunks. Arrange the tofu, tomatoes and herbs in a salad bowl.
   Drizzle over the dressing. Serve with the pepper so that the
   adults can add it at the table.

Beetroot Leaves Salad with Lemon Dressing

When you see beetroots sold with their leafy greens attached,
it is like getting two vegetables for the price of one. I strongly
recommend that you cook and eat both the roots and the leaves.
Cook the leaves just like any other leafy greens like chard, kale
and spinach. Serves 2–4

300g (10½oz) beetroot leaves, stems removed (see Tip)
juice of 1 lemon
1 tsp sugar
a generous pinch of sea salt

1 Bring a large saucepan of water to the boil. Add the beetroot
   leaves and cook over a medium-high heat for 30 seconds.
   Drain and refresh under cold water. Gently squeeze the leaves
   to remove the excess water. Tightly wrap the leaves in kitchen
   paper or muslin and chill in the fridge until ready to use.

2 Put the lemon juice in a small bowl and add the sugar and
   salt. Stir until the sugar and salt dissolve. Unwrap the beetroot
   leaves and cut into 3cm (1¼in) chunks, squeeze out any excess
   water and add to the lemon dressing. Toss well to combine
   and serve immediately.

TIP The beetroot leaf stems can be saved and used for another dish such as a stir-fry or soup.

Main dishes

Donburi Chicken and Eggs Over Fluffy Rice

The word *donburi* means 'medium bowl' and it is also used for a category of stand-alone dishes which are a single medium-sized bowl containing the main dish (protein and vegetables) on top of a bed of rice. Donburi is often served for lunch with a bowl of miso soup and a small side dish. Popular donburi dishes are chicken with eggs, a pork cutlet, prawn and vegetable tempura, and sukiyaki-flavoured thinly sliced beef and vegetables. Serve it with a bowl of soup and a vegetable side dish. Serves 4

4 large eggs
225ml (8fl oz) Dashi Stock (page 182)
1 onion, halved and thinly sliced
1 small leek, cut diagonally into thin slices
½ tsp low-salt, or light, soy sauce
1 tsp sugar
1 tsp salt
1 tsp hon-mirin
225g (8oz) skinless, boneless chicken breasts, cut into bite-sized pieces
1.5kg (3lb 5oz) hot cooked Japanese short-grain rice (white, haiga-mai, or brown) (500g (1lb 2oz) raw weight)
4 mitsuba or flat-leaf parsley sprigs, to garnish

1 Break the eggs into a medium bowl and whisk until just mixed. Put the dashi stock in a medium saucepan over a high heat. Add the onion and leek and bring to the boil. Reduce

the heat to medium and simmer for 5 minutes or until the vegetables are tender.

2   Stir in the soy sauce, sugar, salt and hon-mirin, then add the chicken pieces and cook for 3 minutes.

3   Pour the beaten eggs over the surface of the chicken mixture, so that the egg forms a layer. Reduce the heat to low and cook the mixture for 2 minutes or until the egg and chicken are cooked through. Stir the mixture and turn off the heat. Divide the rice among four bowls and top with the chicken and egg mixture. Garnish each serving with a mitsuba sprig, and serve.

Iri Iri Pan Pan – Super-Scrambled Eggs with Beef, Pork and Mangetout

Every Japanese home chef has her or his own version of this recipe – and children love it because it has three colours: yellow, brown and green. Super-scrambled ingredients make it easy for young children to eat and the different flavours mix well. Serves 4–6

1 tbsp rapeseed, grapeseed or light olive oil
6 large eggs
3 tbsp Dashi Stock (page 182)
1 tbsp sugar
a pinch of salt

For the meat:
1 tbsp rapeseed, grapeseed or light olive oil
200g (7oz) finely ground extra-lean pork (see Tip)
300g (10½oz) finely ground extra-lean beef
2 tsp sugar
1 tbsp reduced-salt soy sauce
130g (4¾oz) mangetouts
500g (1lb 2oz) cooked rice of your choice (140g (5oz) raw weight)

1 Heat the oil in a small saucepan. Mix the eggs, dashi and sugar in a bowl. When the oil is hot, reduce the heat to medium, then add the egg mixture and stir quickly with a wooden cooking fork, or a bundle of three sets of chopsticks, while the egg starts to set. Add a pinch of salt and continue to stir the egg mixture for 2 minutes or until it is just cooked and in very small pieces. Remove the eggs from the pan and set aside.

2 To make the meat, heat the oil in a small saucepan over a high heat. Add the meat, sugar, soy sauce and a pinch of salt to the saucepan, and reduce the heat to medium. Cook the meat, stirring constantly with a wooden cooking fork, or a bundle of three sets of chopsticks, so that it does not clump, for 6 minutes or until cooked through. Remove from the pan and set aside.

3 Put the mangetout in a microwave-safe bowl and heat on full power for 30 seconds. (Alternatively, cook the mangetout in a pan with boiling water to just cover for 4 minutes or until just cooked.) Drain and refresh under cold water. Thinly slice and set aside.

4 Put out four medium bowls for adults, or six small bowls for children. Scoop 2 ladlefuls of the cooked rice for a grown-up, or 1 ladleful for a child, in each bowl. Then gently smooth out the surface with a wet fork, being careful not to squash the rice or pack it too tightly, to make the bed of rice relatively flat. Spoon one-quarter of the super-scrambled eggs for each adult, or one-sixth for a child, over half the rice in each bowl, then add one-quarter of the meat for each adult, or one-sixth for a child, on the other half of the rice. Spread the eggs and meat evenly over their respective sides. Divide the mangetouts among the bowls, where the eggs and meat meet.

5 For young children, you can mix the rice with the meat, eggs and vegetables to make them easier to eat.

TIPS You can use any finely ground meat, or chicken or turkey, of your choice. Ask your butcher to grind it two or three extra times, or grind it again at home in a food processor.

You can use any leftovers from this dish for the Inari Thin Tofu Pouches on page 167.

One-pot Beef, Potato and Onion Casserole

This is a lovely meat and potato dish that is especially appealing in the winter. Serve the casserole at the table with some rice and another vegetable side dish or two. Serves 2–4

  1 tbsp rapeseed oil
  250g (9oz) lean sirloin beef, thinly sliced
  250g (9oz) potatoes, peeled and cut into bite-sized pieces
  2 onions, cut into thin wedges
  2 tbsp low-salt, or light, soy sauce
  a pinch of sea salt

1 Heat the oil in a flameproof casserole or large, heavy-based saucepan over a medium-high heat, and fry the beef for 3 minutes. Remove the beef from the casserole and set aside. Add the potatoes and onions and cook for 5 minutes.

2 Return the beef to the casserole followed by 100ml (3½fl oz) water, the soy sauce and salt. Stir to combine. Partially cover, reduce the heat to medium-low and simmer for 15 minutes or until the potatoes are cooked through, stirring occasionally.

Beef, Mushroom and Vegetable Gyoza Dumplings

Serve these juicy, energy-packed dumplings for children with rice, soup and a tofu or vegetable side dish. It's a fun recipe to make with children. I learned how to make them as a girl standing next to my mum, pinching a gyoza wrapper to close it. The wrappers can be bought from supermarkets or Asian grocers. Serves 4

230g (8oz) lean minced beef
30g (1oz) napa, Chinese or regular cabbage, finely chopped
3 fresh shiitake mushrooms or other mushrooms, stems discarded, caps finely chopped
70g (2½oz) nira (Chinese chives) or chives, finely chopped
2 spring onions, finely chopped
2 tbsp rapeseed, grapeseed or extra virgin olive oil
24 round dumpling wrappers
sea salt and freshly ground black pepper

For the dipping sauce:
50ml (2fl oz) low-salt, or light, soy sauce
50ml (2fl oz) brown rice vinegar
½ tsp sesame oil
shichimi togarashi, or mustard, to serve (optional, for the adults)

1   Put the meat, cabbage, mushrooms, chives and spring onions in a large bowl. Season this filling mixture with a pinch of salt and pepper, if you like. Use your hands to blend the ingredients together.

2   Put a wok or heavy-based frying pan over a high heat. When hot, reduce the heat to medium, add 1 tbsp of the oil and swirl it around to coat the inside of the wok. Add the filling mixture, stir with a spatula, and stir-fry for 5 minutes. Line a baking sheet or large tray with baking parchment.

3   Fill a small bowl with cold water. For each dumpling, put 1 tsp of the filling in the centre of a dumpling wrapper, then lightly dip a finger in the bowl and use it to trace around the inside of the wrapper, which will make it sticky enough to seal.

4   Fold the wrapper in half with the edge on top. Gently press the edges from right to left to seal the dumpling while pinching and folding every 5mm (¼in) of the edge facing you to make a zigzag pattern. Put the dumpling on the prepared baking sheet with the crimped side up, and cover with wet muslin or kitchen paper. Repeat with the remaining dumpling wrappers and filling.

5   To make the dipping sauce, mix the soy sauce, vinegar and oil in a small bowl or jar. Set aside until ready to serve.

6   Put a large frying pan that is deep enough to hold the dumplings over a high heat. Add the remaining oil. When hot, reduce the heat to medium and add the dumplings, crimped side up. Cook the dumplings, uncovered, for 4 minutes or until they are lightly browned underneath.

7   Pour 225ml (8fl oz) water into the frying pan. Cover and steam-cook the dumplings over a medium heat for 8–10 minutes, adding a little more water if needed, until the tops of the dumplings are translucent, the bases are crisp-brown and all the water has evaporated. Serve with the dipping sauce.

TIP You can use other protein, instead of the beef, if you like; for example, a beef–pork mixture – 140g (5oz) beef and 90g (3oz) pork – or pork, chicken, turkey, fish, crab, or prawns.

One-pot Fish with Tofu and Vegetables

This is a seafood version of a one-pot dish: a quick, delicious way to serve protein and vegetables – and it's popular with children, too! Serves 2–4

250g (9oz) white fish fillet, such as cod, tilapia, haddock, whiting), skinned and checked that no small bones remain

200ml Dashi Stock (page 182)
a pinch of sea salt
1 tbsp low-salt, or light, soy sauce
½ carrot, diagonally cut into long 5mm (¼in) thick slices
50g (1¾oz) leek, cut into 5cm (2in) long matchsticks
150g (5½oz) firm tofu, cut into small cubes
10 runner beans, cut into 5cm (2in) long strips
juice of ½ lime, lemon or yuzu, to serve

1   Cut the fish fillet into eight pieces. In a medium flameproof casserole over a medium heat, combine the dashi stock, salt and soy sauce, then add the carrot and leek, and simmer for 3 minutes.

2   Add the tofu, beans and the fish, and simmer for 5 minutes or until the fish is cooked through, skimming the foam from the surface with a ladle. Serve the fish and vegetable mixture in bowls with the sauce spooned over. Serve with the yazu (or lime or lemon) to drizzle over.

TIP Japanese grocers often stock yuzu citrus juice in a bottle. Look for it in the sauce section.

Simmered Bass in Mild Teriyaki Sauce

Cooked in teriyaki sauce, fish fillets will be an appetising caramel-brown colour and taste delicious. Serve it with rice, soup and two side dishes. You can use the teriyaki sauce recipe for other seafood and chicken. Serves 2

2 fillets of sea bass, about 60g (2⅛oz) each
1 tbsp hon-mirin
2 tbsp low-salt, or light, soy sauce
pinch of salt
1 tbsp finely chopped spring onion, to garnish

1   Lay the bass fillets in a shallow saucepan. Add the hon-mirin, soy sauce, salt and 2 tbsp water to the pan and simmer over a medium heat for 4 minutes.

2   Turn the fish over and simmer for 2 minutes or until the fish is cooked through. Transfer the fish to individual shallow bowls and spoon the sauce over the top. Garnish with the spring onion and serve.

Grilled Mackerel

Mackerel is one of Japan's favourites and is packed with omega-3 healthy fats. It is often served grilled as part of a traditional Japanese breakfast but is popular for lunch or dinner as well. As always with fish, but particularly with fish such as mackerel and herrings, be very careful to remove all the small bones before serving to children. Serves 2

> 2 fillets of mackerel, checked for small bones
> 120g (4¼oz) daikon (mooli) or radishes, finely grated and excess liquid drained off (see Tip)
> low-salt, or light, soy sauce, to serve

1   Preheat the grill to medium. Put the fish on the grill pan and cook for 4 minutes. Turn the fish over and cook for 2 minutes or until the centre of one fish flakes when prodded with a sharp knife.

2   Serve with a small amount of grated daikon. Let each diner drizzle a couple of drops of soy sauce over the daikon to flavour it, then eat the daikon with the fish. For young children, flake the fish flesh using a fork, and take out all the bones, making sure that no small bones remain.

TIP If the grated daikon is too spicy for your child, use a sprinkle of lemon juice instead.

Grilled Wild Alaskan Salmon with Broccoli

When wild Alaskan or Pacific salmon is available in the summer, make a point of treating yourself and your family to this melt-in-your-mouth, meaty treasure of the oceans and rivers. Its bright orange-pink colour stands out from the other fish at the fishmonger's. Look for king, chinook, sockeye and coho salmon. When the fish is not in season, use canned or frozen. Serves 2

1 tbsp rapeseed, grapeseed or extra virgin olive oil
½ large onion, halved and thinly sliced
200g (7oz) broccoli florets and stalks
1 tsp hon-mirin
1 tsp low-salt, or light, soy sauce
sea salt and freshly ground black pepper
2 salmon fillets, about 115g (4oz) each
120g (4¼oz) daikon (mooli) or radishes, finely grated, excess liquid drained off, or juice of ½ lemon
2 tbsp shredded nori
2 sprigs of mitsuba or parsley, to garnish
low-salt, or light, soy sauce, to serve

1   Heat the oil in a wok or medium shallow pan over a high heat. Reduce the heat to medium and add the onion. Stir-fry for 5 minutes, then add the broccoli and cook for 3 minutes or until bright green and crisp-tender. Stir in the hon-mirin, soy sauce, 2 tbsp water, the salt and pepper and simmer for 3 minutes. Turn off the heat and set aside.

2   Preheat the grill to high. Reduce the heat to medium and put the fish on the grill rack. Grill for 4 minutes, then turn the fish over and grill for 2 minutes more or until the centre of one fillet flakes when prodded with a sharp knife. Arrange equal portions of the stir-fried vegetables and the grilled salmon on medium-sized plates. Top each serving with a small amount of grated daikon, or a drizzle of lemon juice, the shredded nori

and a mitsuba sprig. Let each diner drizzle a couple of drops of soy sauce over the daikon to flavour it, then eat the daikon with the fish.

Wild Salmon and Asparagus Chahan Fried Rice

Chahan, fried rice, originally from China, is a popular dish, especially among children. All the ingredients are stir-fried, seasoned and mixed, so it is easy and delicious to eat. Chahan is a perfect recipe to use up leftover rice and any odds-and-ends of ingredients left in a fridge. This recipe uses canned salmon. Serve the dish with a light soup. Serves 2

300g (10½oz) asparagus
3 tbsp rapeseed, grapeseed or extra virgin olive oil
2 eggs, beaten
200g (7oz) onion, finely chopped
20g (¾oz) spring onion, finely chopped
a pinch of sea salt (do not add if using salted canned salmon)
½ tsp low-salt, or light, soy sauce
200g (7oz) canned wild Alaskan or sockeye salmon in water, drained
750g (1lb 10oz) cooked Japanese short-grain rice (white, haiga, or brown) (210g (7½oz) raw weight) (page 160)
1 tbsp chopped fresh coriander leaves
freshly ground black pepper

1   Snap off any woody ends from the asparagus stalks at the point where they break easily. Cut the spears into 5mm (¼in) lengths. Set aside.

2   Put a wok or a large, heavy-based frying pan over a high heat. Add 1 tbsp of the oil and swirl it around to coat the wok. When the oil begins to simmer, add the beaten eggs – they will immediately begin to puff in the middle and bubble around the edges. Fry the eggs for 2 minutes, or until the centre portion is

no longer runny. Turn the omelette over and fry for 1 minute more. Transfer to a plate. When the omelette is cool enough to handle, tear it into bite-sized pieces.

3   Heat the remaining oil in the wok, then add the onions and asparagus. Stir-fry for 2 minutes over a medium-high heat. Add the salt, if needed, and the soy sauce. Reduce the heat to medium-high and add the salmon, cooked rice, the torn omelette and the chopped coriander. Use a spatula to crumble the salmon. Toss the ingredients in the wok and stir-fry for 3 minutes, or until the rice and salmon are hot. Serve in medium-sized individual bowls.

Stir-fried Five-colour Veggies with Tofu

Children often like stir-fried vegetables. This dish is colourful and tasty, and has the added protein of tofu. Serves 2

1 tbsp rapeseed, grapeseed or extra virgin olive oil
1 onion, sliced
2 garlic cloves, crushed
50g (1¾oz) shallots, finely chopped
120g (4¼oz) carrots, sliced diagonally 5mm (¼in) thick
¼ head of broccoli, broken into bite-sized florets
250g (9oz) courgette, sliced diagonally 5mm (¼in) thick
2 tbsp Sweet Dashi–Soy Seasoning Sauce (page 184)
100g (3½oz) extra-firm tofu, rinsed and cut into 2.5cm (1in) cubes
1 red pepper, deseeded and thinly sliced
1 tsp toasted sesame oil
2 coriander sprigs, to garnish
freshly ground black pepper (optional, for the adults)

1   Heat the oil in a wok or large frying pan over a high heat. Reduce the heat to medium and add the onion, garlic, shallots and carrots. Stir-fry for 3 minutes. Add the broccoli and stir-fry for 3 minutes. Add the courgette. Continue stir-frying

the vegetables for 3 minutes or until the carrots are cooked through and crisp-tender.

2   Stir in 100ml (3½fl oz) water and the sweet dashi–soy seasoning sauce, and cook for 3 minutes. Add the tofu and red pepper, toss to mix and stir-fry for 2 minutes, or until most of the seasoning liquid has evaporated. Drizzle the sesame oil all over, toss to mix and turn off the heat. Transfer to a large serving bowl and garnish with coriander. Serve with the pepper, if you like.

Donburi Japanese Sweet Potato and Vegetables Over Sushi Rice

The sweet flavours of the sweet potatoes and veggies mingle deliciously with the vinegar in the sushi rice. Serve this dish with a protein side dish and a soup. Serves 2

2 dried shiitake mushrooms
2 tbsp low-salt, or light, soy sauce
1 tbsp hon-mirin
a pinch of sea salt
150g (5½oz) Japanese sweet potato (bushbok, white flesh, kumara, or use regular sweet potato), peeled and cut into 1cm (½in) cubes
200g (7oz) carrots, finely chopped
100g (3½oz) celery, finely chopped
50g (1¾oz) leek, cut into 3mm (⅛in) thick slices
750g (1lb 10oz) cooked vinegared rice (210g (7½oz) raw weight) (page 162)
10g (¼oz) Toasted Ground White Sesame Seeds (page 186)

1   Put the shiitake mushrooms in a small bowl and add 100ml (3½fl oz) water. Leave to soak for 20 minutes. Strain the soaking water into a small bowl, then blend in the soy sauce, the hon-mirin and salt. Squeeze the mushrooms gently to remove the excess water, then cut off and discard the stems. Finely chop the caps.

2   Put the sweet potato in a medium saucepan and add the carrots, celery, leek, mushrooms and the shiitake liquid. Simmer
over a medium heat for 15 minutes or until the vegetables are
cooked through. (Alternatively, put the vegetables and dashi
mixture into a microwavable steamer and microwave on full
power for 2 minutes, or according to the steamer/microwave
instructions.)

3   Fill each serving bowl with half the vinegared rice and arrange
even portions of the simmered vegetables over the top. Garnish each serving with a sprinkling of the sesame seeds.

Vegetable Gyoza Dumplings

These vegetarian dumplings are a delicious way to increase the
vegetable intake for families with young children. They also make
a lovely party platter if you have vegetarian guests. Serves 4

100g/4oz pearl barley
75g (2¾oz) cabbage, finely chopped
75g (2¾oz) carrots, grated
5 fresh shiitake mushrooms, stems discarded and caps finely
chopped, or chestnut mushrooms, chopped
45g (1½oz) nira (Chinese chives) or garlic chives, chives or
shallots, finely chopped
2 spring onions, finely chopped
2 tbsp rapeseed, grapeseed or extra virgin olive oil
24 round gyoza dumpling wrappers
sea salt and freshly ground black pepper
shichimi togarashi, or mustard, to serve (optional, for the
adults)

For the dipping sauce:
50ml (2fl oz) low-salt, or light, soy sauce
50ml (2fl oz) brown rice vinegar
½ tsp sesame oil

1 Cook the barley in a saucepan of boiling water for 30 minutes, or according to the package instructions, until tender.
Drain and set aside. Put the cabbage, carrots, mushrooms,
chives and spring onions in a large bowl, and season with
several generous pinches of salt. Use your hands to blend the
ingredients together.

2 Put a wok or a heavy-based frying pan over a high heat. When
hot, reduce the heat to medium, add 1 tbsp of the oil and swirl
it around to coat the inside of the wok. Add the vegetable
mixture and stir with a spatula. Stir-fry for 5 minutes. Turn off
the heat, add the barley, and toss to mix. Line a baking sheet
with baking parchment.

3 Fill a small bowl with cold water. For each dumpling, put 1
tsp of filling in the centre of a gyoza wrapper. Lightly wet one
finger in the water and trace around the inside of the gyoza
wrapper, which will make it sticky enough to seal.

4 Fold the wrapper in half, with the edge on top. Gently press
the edges from right to left to seal the dumpling while pinching and folding every 5mm (¼in) of the edge facing you to
make a zigzag pattern. Put the completed dumplings on the
prepared baking sheet with the crimped side up, and cover
with damp kitchen paper to prevent them from drying. Repeat
with the remaining dumpling wrappers and filling.

5 To make the dipping sauce, mix the soy sauce, vinegar and oil
in a small bowl. Set aside.

6 Put a large frying pan that is deep enough to hold the dumplings over a high heat. Add the remaining oil. When hot,
reduce the heat to medium and add the dumplings, crimped
side up. Cook the dumplings, uncovered, for 4 minutes or
until they are lightly browned underneath.

7 Pour 225ml (8fl oz) water into the frying pan. Cover and
steam-cook the dumplings over a medium heat for 8–10
minutes, adding a little more water if needed, until the tops of

the dumplings are translucent, the bases are crisp-brown and all the water has evaporated. Serve with the dipping sauce and shichimi togarashi, if you like.

TIP Instead of frying the dumplings, you can steam them in a steamer for 15 minutes or in a microwave steamer for 5 minutes, or until the filling is cooked through.

Rice

Fluffy Japanese Short-Grain Rice

Makes 650g (1lb 7oz) about 4 rice bowls

Stove-top method

300g (10½oz) short-grain white rice, or haiga-mai, or short-grain brown rice

1 Do not rinse haiga-mai rice. Some brands of white and brown rice do not require washing, so please read the directions on the packet. Otherwise, if using white or brown rice, wash the rice by putting the grains in a medium bowl and adding cold water to cover. Swish the grains with your hand to remove the starch and then drain off the cloudy water by tilting the bowl and holding the rice in the bowl with your cupped palm. Repeat this process two or three more times, or until the water, when agitated around the rice, is almost clear. Drain the rice in a fine-meshed sieve.

2 Put the rice in a medium saucepan. Add 340ml (12fl oz) water for white rice or haiga-mai, or 410ml (14½fl oz) for brown rice, and leave the rice to soak for 20 minutes for white and haiga-mai, and 60 minutes – or longer, even overnight – for brown rice, until plump.

3   Cover the saucepan and bring the rice to the boil. Reduce the heat to low and gently simmer for 15 minutes for white or haiga-mai rice, or 30 minutes for brown rice, or until all the liquid has evaporated. Turn off the heat, cover and leave the rice to stand for 10 minutes. When ready to serve, fluff up the rice by gently turning it over with a wet wooden or plastic rice paddle or spoon.

4   You can cook rice ahead of time, leave it to cool to room temperature and portion it into single-serve freezer-proof containers, and freeze. Defrost in the microwave in a microwave-safe container, loosely covered.

Electric rice cooker method

300g (10½oz) short-grain white rice, or haiga-mai, or short-grain brown rice

1   Wash the rice as for the stove-top method. Transfer the rice to the cooking bowl of an electric rice cooker. Add water to the bowl according to the manufacturer's instructions. Set the cooking mode according to the type of rice you're cooking, either white, haiga-mai or brown rice. Leave the rice to soak for 20 minutes for white and haiga-mai, and 60 minutes – or longer, even overnight – for brown rice, until plump, then turn on the rice cooker. The cooker automatically turns off when it's done (about 20–30 minutes, depending on the model). When the rice has finished cooking, leave it to rest undisturbed for 10 minutes without opening the lid. When ready to serve, fluff up the rice by gently turning it over with a wet wooden or plastic rice paddle or spoon.

Onigiri Rice Balls

These rice balls are Japan's ancient on-the-go snacks and meals for picnics, days out and lunch boxes. Makes 6

85g (3oz) wild Alaskan salmon fillet or king, chinook, sockeye or coho salmon
400g (14oz) cooked Japanese short-grain rice (white or haiga-mai), or rice-barley-mixed (110g (3¾oz) raw weight) (see pages 160 and 164)
6 nori sheets (3 × 10cm/1¼ × 4in)

1 Preheat the grill to medium. Put the salmon on the grill rack and grill for 6–7 minutes until the salmon is just cooked through. Leave to cool. Remove the skin from the salmon and break the salmon into six pieces.

2 Lightly wet both hands in a small bowl of water to prevent the grains from sticking to your palms. Put a small handful of rice in one hand and use the thumb of your other hand to make a deep indentation in the centre of the rice.

3 Put one piece of salmon in the indentation and then cover it over with the rice. Lightly squeeze both hands around the rice to shape it into a round, rotating and gently squeezing the rice a couple of times until it becomes well packed and solid. Repeat the process with the other pieces of salmon, dipping your hands into the bowl of water between making each ball.

4 Wrap a sheet of nori around each ball and serve.

TIP Shortcut: use canned low-salt Alaskan salmon.

Vinegared Rice for Sushi, aka Sushi Rice

Use this rice to make sushi rolls, inari sushi (page 167) and sushi dishes (pages 157, 164, 165). Serves 4

1 piece dried kombu, 10cm (4in) square
400g/14oz short-grain rice, either haiga-mai, white or mixed
2 tbsp and 1 tsp brown rice vinegar

2 tbsp sugar

1 tsp salt

1 tsp hon-mirin

1 Soak the kombu in 500ml (18fl oz) water for about 1 hour to make a cooking stock. Rinse the rice according to the package instructions and drain in a sieve, then set aside for at least 30 minutes and preferably 60 minutes.

2 Combine the vinegar, sugar, salt and hon-mirin in a small pan, and heat gently to dissolve the sugar. Set aside. Put the stock and rice into a rice cooker and leave it to soak for 10–15 minutes until plump, then set the cooker to either sushi or regular white rice cooking mode, and turn it on. The cooker automatically turns off when it's done (about 20–30 minutes, depending on the model). (Alternatively, for cooking in a pan, put the stock and rice in a medium saucepan with a tight-fitting lid, and leave it to soak for 10–15 minutes until plump, then follow the stove-top method for cooking rice on page 160.) When finished, leave it to rest undisturbed for 10 minutes without opening the lid.

3 Moisten a shallow wooden sushi rice tub, or large casserole, with vinegar water (see Tip) so that the cooked grains will not stick, and transfer the grains to the tub. Fluff up the grains by gently turning them over with a wet rice paddle or spoon.

4 Sprinkle the vinegar dressing over the rice. Gently toss the rice using horizontal cutting strokes with the paddle or spoon, so as not to squash the grains, while cooling the rice using a hand fan or by waving a sheet of plastic or cardboard over it. Cover with a clean cloth moistened with vinegar water.

TIP To make vinegar water for the hands, rice tub and knives when making sushi, add 2 tbsp rice vinegar to 250ml (9fl oz) water. Make more of this solution if needed.

Vinegared Rice-barley For Sushi

I created this recipe so that I could incorporate barley into some of our meals. Use this rice to make sushi rolls, inari sushi (page 167) and sushi dishes (pages 157, 165). Makes 950g (2lb 2oz)

1 kombu sheet, 10cm (4in) square
200g (7oz) short-grain white rice
100g (3½oz) haiga-mai short-grain rice
100g (3½oz) pot or pearl barley
4 tbsp brown rice vinegar
2 tbsp sugar
1 tsp salt
1 tsp hon-mirin

Follow the Vinegared Rice for Sushi, aka Sushi Rice recipe (page 162).

Hosomaki (Skinny Sushi Roll)

Because sushi rolls are so popular and almost synonymous with Japanese food outside of Japan, I believe that making them at home can be a wonderful gateway for your child to have fun and be exposed to a Japanese-style meal. Sushi rolls, just like onigiri rice balls, are the equivalent of Western sandwiches and make a fantastic stand-alone meal served with soup, or a healthy delicious snack. You can pack them in a lunch-box or take them to a picnic. They also make a lovely party platter. Experiment with a variety of fillings and enjoy! Makes 1 roll

vinegar water, see Tip page 163
1 sheet of nori
80g (2¾oz) cooked Sushi Rice (25g (1oz) raw weight) (page 162)
½ tsp wasabi (optional, for the adults)

40–60g (1½–2⅛oz) fillings of your choice, such as cooked
seafood, grated carrot, cucumber cut into thin matchsticks,
¼ avocado, sliced
low-salt soy sauce, to serve

1 Make up the vinegar water. Put a completely dry bamboo
sushi mat on your work surface, with the bamboo sticks running horizontally. Put the nori, rough-side up, horizontally
on the mat. Moisten your palms with the vinegar water, put
the rice on the nori sheet, and gently spread the rice with
moistened fingertips so as not to squash the grains. Spread
the rice evenly over the entire nori sheet except for the top
1cm (½in) with your fingertips moistened with the vinegar
water. Spread the wasabi, if using, horizontally in the centre
of the rice bed.

2 Layer the fillings evenly and horizontally on top of the wasabi
in the centre of the rice bed. Lift and roll the mat from the
edge closest to you, gently pushing the fillings in place using
the fingertips, meeting the front edge to the top of the rice
bed, and creating a circular log shape.

3 Put the sushi roll on a dry chopping board horizontally, and
cut the log into six equal parts with a sharp knife moistened
with a vinegar-watered kitchen cloth. Wipe the knife with the
cloth each time you slice. Serve with a small dish of the soy
sauce.

Futomaki (Thick Sushi Roll)

These thick sushi rolls are more substantial than the thin versions. Use protein and vegetable ingredients for the filling. Makes
1 roll

vinegar water, see Tip page 163
1 sheet of nori
120g (4¼oz) Sushi Rice (35g (1¼oz) raw weight) (page 162)

2 teaspoons Toasted and Ground White Sesame Seeds (page 186)
½ tsp wasabi (optional, for the adults)
60–80g (2⅛–3oz) fillings of your choice, such as 50g (1¾oz) salmon, 20g (¾oz) grated carrot, cucumber cut into thin matchsticks, ¼ avocado, sliced
low-salt soy sauce, to serve

1 Make up the vinegar water. Wrap the bamboo sushi mat with clingfilm, or put it in a zip-lock bag, so that the rice won't stick to the mat. Put the mat on the work surface, with the bamboo sticks running horizontally. Put the nori, rough-side up, horizontally on the mat. Moisten your palms with the vinegar water, put the rice on the nori sheet, and spread the rice with moistened fingertips gently so as not to squash the grains. Spread the rice evenly over the entire nori sheet except the top 1cm (½in) with your fingertips moistened with the vinegar water.

2 Sprinkle the sesame seeds evenly over the rice. Flip the nori and rice over, so that the nori sheet now faces you, with the rice bed underneath. Spread the wasabi, if using, horizontally in the centre of the nori–rice bed.

3 Layer the fillings evenly and horizontally on top of the wasabi in the centre of the nori–rice bed. Lift and roll the mat from the edge closest to you, gently pushing the fillings in place using the fingertips, meeting the front edge to the top of the rice bed, and creating a circular log shape.

4 Put the sushi roll horizontally on a dry chopping board, and cut the log into six equal parts with a sharp knife moistened with a vinegar-watered kitchen cloth. Wipe the knife with the cloth each time you slice. Serve with a small dish of the soy sauce.

Inari Thin Tofu Pouches filled with Sushi Rice

Along with onigiri rice balls, these little tofu pouches are staples in lunch boxes and at picnics in Japan. The thin, deep-fried tofu pouches are cooked in sweet soya dashi sauce, making it a delightful portable lunch or snack, especially for those children (and grown-ups) who love 'sweet' flavoured foods. Inari pouches are available at Japanese grocers. Makes 12 pouches

190g (6¾oz) vinegared rice (55g (2oz) raw weight) (page 162)
2 tbsp Toasted and Ground White Sesame Seeds (page 186)
75ml (2½fl oz/⅓ cup) measure of super-scrambled eggs with minced meat or fish (page 147)
12 inari (seasoned deep-fried thin tofu) pouches

1 In a large bowl, mix the vinegared rice, sesame seeds and super-scrambled eggs with meat. Toss them using a wet spatula or rice paddle to mix, being careful not to squash the rice grains.

2 Divide the vinegared rice mixture into 12 portions. Open an inari pouch by gently separating the two sides of the tofu as you would to open a pitta bread. Moisten the palms of your hands with vinegar water (page 163), then gently make a loose oval-shaped rice ball and insert it into the inari pouch. Fold over the loose edge to close. Serve at room temperature.

Rice with Edamame

Serve this protein-rich edamame rice instead of plain rice for a meal, for breakfast, lunch or dinner with a bowl of soup and two or three protein and vegetable dishes. If you cannot find edamame, use peas. If you can find fresh edamame in season, on the other hand, it will make a lovely bowl of rice during the summer!

370g (13oz) Japanese short-grain white rice or haiga-mai
225g (8oz) fresh shelled edamame beans, or frozen shelled
edamame beans, or green peas

1 Wash the rice according to the instructions on page 160. To
   cook the rice, put it in a medium pan. Add 570ml (20fl oz)
   water and leave the rice to soak for 20 minutes until plump.

2 Add the edamame on top of the rice, but do not mix it in.
   Cover the pan and bring the rice to the boil. Reduce the heat
   to low and simmer the rice gently for 15 minutes or until all
   the liquid has evaporated. Turn off the heat, cover and leave
   the rice to stand for 10 minutes. When ready to serve, fluff
   up the rice and edamame by gently turning it over with a wet
   wooden or plastic rice paddle or spoon.

Noodles

Soba Noodles with Sardines and Spinach

Canned sardines are very cheap and nutritious, and a useful food
to have in the storecupboard. The flavour of fatty fish blends well
with the nutty soba buckwheat and the broth. Serves 4

500g (1lb 2oz) spinach, stems removed
1 litre (1¾ pints) Dashi Stock (page 182)
50ml (2fl oz) hon-mirin
50ml low-salt, or light, soy sauce
1 tsp sugar
1 tsp salt
450g (1lb) dried soba (buckwheat noodles)
120g (4¼oz) can boneless sardine fillets, drained
1 spring onion, thinly sliced and 4 tiny mitsuba or flat-leaf
parsley sprigs, to garnish
shichimi togarashi (dried seven-spice chilli), to serve for the
adults

1 Bring a large saucepan of water to the boil. Add the spinach leaves and cook over a medium-high heat for 30 seconds. Drain and refresh under cold water. Gently squeeze the leaves to remove the excess water. Tightly wrap the leaves in kitchen paper or muslin and chill in the fridge until ready to use.

2 Put the dashi stock in a large saucepan over a high heat and stir in the hon-mirin, soy sauce, sugar and salt. Bring the mixture just to the boil, then reduce the heat to very low and keep the mixture warm.

3 Put a large saucepan of water over a high heat. Add the noodles and stir to prevent sticking. Cook the noodles for 6–8 minutes, or according to the packet instructions, until just cooked through. Drain and rinse in a colander under cold water to remove any residual starch.

4 Unroll the tea towel with the spinach, squeeze out any excess water from the leaves and cut the spinach into 2.5cm (1in) pieces.

5 Bring the stock mixture back to the boil. Divide the noodles among four large soup bowls. Lay a small mound of spinach and a sardine fillet over the noodles and cover with the broth mixture. Garnish each serving with spring onion and a sprig of mitsuba. Serve with the shichimi togarashi so that the adults can add it at the table to season their food.

Cool Summer Soba Noodle Salad

In summer, people in Japan often eat cool noodle dishes to ward off the heat and fatigue. Serve the dish at room temperature, not cold from the fridge. This recipe can be used for other types of noodles explained in 'Discovering Japanese Ingredients' on page 126. Serves 2

125ml (4fl oz) Dashi Stock (page 182)
5 tsp hon-mirin
5 tsp low-salt, or light, soy sauce

200g (7oz) dried soba (buckwheat noodles)
a handful of ice cubes in a bowl of cold water
2 large eggs
120g (4¼oz) firm tofu, drained and roughly chopped
2 tbsp rapeseed oil
1 onion, halved and thinly sliced
2 garlic cloves, crushed

For the garnish:
1 spring onion, chopped
1 tbsp sesame or flaxseeds, dry-toasted (page 186)
1 tbsp chopped fresh shiso (optional)
1 tbsp chopped fresh basil leaves
½ tsp freshly grated wasabi, or shop-bought wasabi for the
adults (optional)

1 Put the dashi stock in a small saucepan over a high heat and
   add the hon-mirin and soy sauce. Bring to the boil, turn off
   the heat and leave to cool to room temperature. (To speed
   up cooling, put the mixture in a small metal bowl, nestle
   the small metal bowl in a larger bowl half-filled with ice and
   water, and stir the sauce occasionally.)

2 Put a large saucepan of water over a high heat and bring to
   the boil. Add the noodles and stir to prevent sticking. Cook
   the noodles for 6–8 minutes or according to the packet
   instructions, until just cooked through. Drain the soba in a
   colander and rinse under cold water to remove any residual
   starch. Just before serving, drench the noodles in iced water
   to tighten them, then drain.

3 Put the eggs into a food processor or blender and add the tofu.
   Blend until smooth. Heat 1 tbsp oil in a medium frying pan
   over a medium-high heat. When the oil is hot, stir in the egg
   and tofu mixture. Fry the mixture for 3 minutes or until the
   underneath is golden. Turn the egg-tofu omelette over and fry
   for 2 minutes more or until the underneath is golden brown.

Transfer the omelette to a chopping board and cut into eight pieces. Set aside to cool.

4   Heat the remaining oil in a frying pan over a medium heat. When the oil is hot, add the onion and garlic, and cook for 3 minutes or until the onions are translucent. Set aside to cool. Serve the noodles in bowls and top with the onion and garlic, and the egg mixture, then pour the dashi sauce over the top. Let the diners garnish their meals at the table with the spring onion, seeds, shiso, if using, basil leaves and wasabi, if using.

TIP You can buy ready-made dipping sauce, to use instead of the sauce in the recipe, at specialist Japanese grocers or grocers who stock international condiments. The sauces are usually marked 'dipping sauce for noodles – ready to use soba tsuyu', or similar, on the label.

Kitsune Udon

This is a very basic bowl of udon white wheat noodles topped with thin, deep-fried tofu, which you can find at Japanese grocery stores. It's typically a child's favourite noodle dish. It warms you up on cold days and it makes a quick lunch. Serve it with a vegetable side dish. Serves 4

2 usu-age (thin-fried) tofu
1 litre (1¾ pints) Dashi Stock (page 182)
50ml (2fl oz) hon-mirin
50ml (2fl oz) low-salt, or light, soy sauce
1 tsp sugar
1 tsp salt
450g (1lb) udon noodles
1 chopped spring onion and 1 tbsp Toasted and Ground White Sesame Seeds or flaxseeds (page 186), to garnish

1 Bring a small saucepan of water to the boil. Add the usu-age tofu and gently simmer it over a medium heat, turning occasionally, for 1 minute (this will remove the excess oil). Drain. When cool, squeeze out the excess water, and slice into 1cm (½in) strips. Set aside.

2 To make noodle broth, put the dashi stock in a large saucepan over a high heat and stir in the hon-mirin, soy sauce, sugar and salt. Bring the mixture just to the boil, then reduce the heat to very low and keep the mixture warm.

3 Put a large saucepan of water over a high heat and bring to the boil. Add the noodles and stir to prevent sticking. Cook the noodles for 5–6 minutes or according to the packet instructions, until just cooked through. Drain and put an equal portion of noodles topped with the usu-age tofu slices in a deep bowl. Pour the hot broth over the noodles and tofu slices. Garnish with the spring onion and sesame seeds.

Side dishes

Scrambled Tofu with Salmon

This is a quick-to-make, wonderful protein dish. Serve it with rice, soup and vegetable dishes. Serves 2

200g (7oz) firm tofu, rinsed
1 tbsp rapeseed, grapeseed or extra virgin olive oil
50g (1¾oz) canned Alaskan salmon in water, drained
a pinch of sea salt
2 tbsp Sweet Dashi–Soy Seasoning Sauce (page 184)
freshly ground black pepper for adults (optional)
3 finely chopped spring onions, to garnish

1 Wrap the tofu in two layers of kitchen paper or muslin, put in a microwave-safe container and microwave for 3 minutes.

(Alternatively, wrap the tofu in kitchen paper or muslin and squeeze it by hand to release the water.)

2   Heat the oil in a medium saucepan over a high heat. When the oil is hot, reduce the heat to medium, add the tofu and break it up into rough chunks using a spoon or spatula. Add the salmon and break it up into rough chunks, combining them with the tofu chunks. Sprinkle over the salt and pepper and seasoning sauce. Turn off the heat. Serve the tofu and salmon hot, garnished with spring onions.

Sardines and Cherry Tomatoes

Cooking fish in oil diminishes its fishiness and makes it more enjoyable for children to eat. Keep some cans of sardines in the storecupboard to make omega-3-rich meals that take moments to prepare. Cherry tomatoes are sweet and juicy, and can be eaten for a snack as well. Serves 2

    1 tbsp rapeseed, grapeseed or extra virgin olive oil
    120g (4¼oz) can sardines in water, drained
    10 cherry tomatoes, halved
    1 spring onion, chopped
    ½ lemon, cut into two wedges, to serve
    sea salt and freshly ground black pepper

1   Heat the oil in a small, non-stick frying pan over a high heat. Reduce the heat to medium-high and add the sardines. Add a pinch of salt and black pepper and cook for 2 minutes.

2   Add the tomatoes and spring onion, and gently cook for 2 minutes. Serve with lemon for squeezing over the fish.

Simmered Daikon and Tofu

As daikon slowly absorbs the broth, its natural sweet flavour mingles with the broth, creating a delightful sensation that bursts and melts in your mouth. Tofu is more subtle and softer. Serves 4

400g (14oz) daikon (mooli), cut into bite-sized pieces
600ml (20fl oz) Dashi Stock (page 182)
1 tsp sea salt
1 tsp sugar
1 tsp low-salt, or light, soy sauce
250g (9oz) firm tofu, rinsed and cut into bite-sized cubes

1 Put the daikon and dashi stock in a medium saucepan over a medium-high heat and bring to the boil. Reduce the heat to medium-low and stir in the salt, sugar and soy sauce. Partially cover and simmer for 50 minutes, stirring occasionally, or until the daikon has absorbed two-thirds of the liquid.

2 Add the tofu and simmer for 10 minutes or until the daikon and tofu have absorbed almost all the liquid. Transfer to a serving bowl.

Aubergines and Red Peppers with Sweet Red Miso Sauce

Japanese aubergines are long and thin. Besides the shape, one important difference between Japanese aubergines and those of the UK and the US is that their flesh is denser and meatier. Try to find locally grown Japanese aubergines if you can. Otherwise, Mediterranean aubergines have similar features.

To make the dish child-friendly, I use red (or orange or yellow) peppers for their sweetness and bright appetising colour on the plate. The aubergines' soft meaty texture contrasts well with the peppers' crunchiness. Children love them wrapped in a savoury-sweet miso sauce. Serves 4

450g (1lb) Japanese or Mediterranean aubergines, peeled and cut into bite-sized pieces
225ml (8fl oz) rapeseed oil
2 red (or orange and/or yellow) peppers, deseeded and cut into bite-sized pieces
4 tsp Sweet Red Miso Sauce (page 187)

1 tsp Toasted and Ground White Sesame Seeds (page 186)
½ tsp toasted sesame oil

1   Put the aubergine pieces in a bowl of water and leave them to soak for 5 minutes. Drain and thoroughly wipe off the excess water with kitchen paper.

2   Heat the oil in a wok or large, deep frying pan over a medium heat until it reaches 180°C/350°F on a cooking thermometer. (Alternatively, test the oil with a cube of fresh bread; if the bread rises to the surface and immediately turns golden, the oil is hot enough.)

3   Carefully slip the aubergine pieces into the oil. Fry for 3 minutes, adjusting the heat as necessary to keep the oil temperature at around 180°C/350°F. Rotate and fry the aubergine on all sides for 1–2 minutes more or until the flesh is soft. Test for doneness by piercing the flesh with a wooden skewer: you should be able to slide it easily all the way through.

4   Transfer the aubergine to a rack lined with a double layer of kitchen paper to drain them. Pour off the oil from the wok into a metal container (to discard or use on another occasion).

5   The wok will still be coated with a small amount of oil. Put the wok over a medium-high heat and add the peppers. Stir-fry for 2 minutes or until the pepper is bright red. Add the aubergine pieces and the sweet miso sauce and gently toss the vegetables to coat with the sauce. Transfer to a serving dish and sprinkle with the sesame seeds and sesame oil.

Steamed Veggies with Lemon-Soy Sauce

These vegetables are served with a sprinkling of lemon juice and soy sauce, plus some ginger for the adults. Those simple seasonings make plain vegetables very tasty and more appealing to children (and adults). Serves 4

200g (7oz) potatoes, peeled, cut into bite-sized pieces
1 onion, halved and sliced
200g (7oz) green, orange and yellow peppers, deseeded and
sliced into strips
300g (10½oz) courgettes, sliced
300g (10½oz) yellow courgettes or patty pan squash, sliced

To serve:
juice of 2 lemons
low-salt, or light, soy sauce
1cm (½in) fresh root ginger, peeled and finely grated, for the
adults

1   Put the potatoes and onion in a steamer over boiling
    water and cook for 10 minutes over a medium heat, add
    the peppers and continue to steam for 5 minutes, then
    add the courgettes and steam for 5 more minutes or until
    the potatoes are cooked through and the other vegetables
    are crisp-tender. (Alternatively, in a microwave steamer,
    microwave the vegetables for 1–3 minutes on full power,
    until crisp-tender, or according to the steamer/microwave
    instructions.)

2   Serve the vegetables with lemon juice and soy sauce to be
    added at the table, with ginger for the adults.

Tender Vegetables with Sweet Sesame Dressing

Spinach marinated in a sweet, white sesame dressing is a frequent
side dish in a home-made Japanese meal and at many Japanese
restaurants around the world. This dish, because it is sweet-
flavoured, is often a young child's favourite. Use it for any variety
of vegetables. Serves 4

500g (1lb 2oz) vegetables, such as broccoli, cauliflower,
radish, carrots, asparagus, runner beans or green beans, cut
into small bite-sized pieces or matchsticks, and leafy greens

(baby spinach, kale, spring greens or chard), left as whole
leaves
2½ tbsp Sweet White Sesame Seed Soy Sauce Dressing
(page 187)

1   Put the vegetables in a steamer over boiling water and cook
for 5 minutes for all vegetables except the leafy greens or
until crisp-tender, and 3 minutes for leafy greens or until just
wilted. (Alternatively, in a microwave steamer, microwave
the vegetables except the leafy greens for 2–3 minutes on full
power and the leafy greens for 1–2 minutes – or according to
the steamer/microwave instructions). Immediately run the
vegetables under cold water to prevent them from further
cooking.

2   Drain and gently squeeze the leafy greens to release the excess
water. Cut the greens into 1cm (½in) pieces and put them in a
serving bowl. Pour over the sesame dressing and mix well. Add
the other vegetables and mix to combine.

Steamed Japanese Sweet Potatoes

When I was growing up in Japan, Japanese sweet potatoes were
such a big part of the diet that sweet potato wagons would
come to our neighbourhood of Tokyo offering the vegetable as
an afternoon snack during the winter. But more often, mum
steamed loads of them and left them out on a table for us to
enjoy. Serves 4

1 large or 2 medium Japanese sweet potatoes (bushbok,
white flesh or use regular sweet potatoes), about 1kg (2lb
4oz), unpeeled and cut into 2cm (¾in) thick rounds

1   Bring 3 litres (5¼ pints) water to the boil in a large steamer or
saucepan. Add the sweet potatoes to the steamer or to a colander over the pan, cover and steam over a medium-high heat

for 20 minutes, or until the potatoes are cooked through. Test by piercing the flesh with a wooden skewer: it should slide easily all the way through. (Alternatively, put the potatoes in a microwave steamer, close the lid with a vent open, and cook for 3–5 minutes on full power, until cooked through.) Serve hot or at room temperature. The cooked potatoes will keep in an airtight plastic bag in the fridge for up to three days.

Baked Japanese Sweet Potato Sticks

I decided to make tastier and more nutritious snacks than shop-bought or restaurant-served French fries for my son. The sweet potato, especially the Japanese variety, is the champion of vegetables – packed with nutrition – as I explained earlier, and it tastes great cut into sticks and baked. I keep the skin on to preserve the most nutritious part, which is between the skin and the flesh, and to give the sticks an extra-hearty, authentic touch. Serves 4–6

> 1 large or 2 medium Japanese sweet potatoes (bushbok, white flesh, kumara or use regular sweet potato), about 1kg (2lb 4oz), unpeeled
> 1 tbsp rapeseed, grapeseed or extra virgin olive oil

1   Preheat the oven to 220°C/425°F/Gas 7. Cut the potato into 5cm (2in) long sticks, 1cm (½in) wide, then rinse in cold water, changing the water two to three times, until it is almost clear. Drain the potato, and pat it dry with kitchen paper.

2   Transfer the potato to a bowl, pour the oil over and toss well. Spread the potato sticks on a non-stick baking sheet in a single layer, leaving space between them. Bake for 20 minutes, then turn them over and bake for another 15–20 minutes or until golden brown. Transfer the baking sheet to a cooling rack. Serve the sticks warm or at room temperature.

Baked Japanese Sweet Potatoes

An anytime, anywhere, almighty snack and side dish. Serves 4–6

> 1 large, or 2 medium Japanese sweet potatoes (bushbok, white flesh, kumara or use regular sweet potato) about 1kg (2lb 4oz), unpeeled

1   Preheat the oven to 180°C/350°F/Gas 4. Put the sweet potato on a baking sheet. Bake a large sweet potato for 1½ hours and a medium sweet potato for 1 hour, turning it over once halfway through. Test for doneness by piercing the flesh with a wooden skewer: you should be able to slide it easily all the way through. Break open the sweet potato immediately to let the steam out and to avoid it becoming mushy. (Alternatively, microwave a sweet potato for 6 minutes on full power – or according to the steamer/microwave instructions – then remove it from the microwave and immediately wrap it in foil. Leave it to rest for 2 minutes.)

Sautéed Beetroot

Serve this as a side dish in autumn with your choice of fish, meat, poultry, soya, pulse and/or other vegetable dish. Beetroot is so naturally sweet that no seasoning is necessary. It is a lovely side dish for the late autumn. Serves 2

> 1 tbsp rapeseed, grapeseed or extra virgin olive oil
> 3 small beetroots, peeled and sliced into 5mm (¼in) thick rounds

1   Heat a large frying pan and add the oil. Cook the beetroot over a medium-high heat for 5 minutes or until crisp on the outside and all the liquid has evaporated from the pan. Transfer the beetroot to a rack lined with a double layer of kitchen paper to drain the excess oil. Serve hot.

Oven-roasted Super-sweet Beetroot

Amazingly sweet, ruby-red beetroots make a trophy snack. The oven-roasting method helps intensify the natural sugar in the beetroot as it does to sweet potatoes. Beetroot contains fibre and potassium and is an excellent source of folate. Our son popped these cube-shaped beetroots into his mouth when he started feeding himself. Serves 4

> 500g (1lb 2oz) beetroot, peeled and cut into 1cm (½in) cubes
> 2 tbsp rapeseed, grapeseed or extra virgin olive oil

1   Preheat the oven to 220°C/425°F/Gas 7. Put the beetroot in a large bowl and toss with the oil to coat. Spread the cubes in a single layer in a roasting pan and roast for 25–40 minutes until tender, turning twice. Remove the tray from the oven and allow to cool a little before serving.

Lightly Simmered Crudités with Creamy Tofu and Chickpea Dipping Sauce

These are ideal first finger foods, because they are soft enough for babies to eat to move on from puréed food to solids. Young children love to dip. Let them have fun with this creamy protein-rich sauce. Serves 4

> a handful of ice cubes
> 1 carrot, cut into 5cm (2in) long sticks
> ¼ cauliflower head, cut into small florets with stems
> 1 red pepper, seeded and cut into strips
> 1 yellow pepper, seeded, and cut into strips
> 8 sugar snap peas, trimmed
> 250g (9oz) daikon (mooli) radish cut into 5cm (2in) sticks, or white turnip sliced into wedges

8 cherry tomatoes
salt
Creamy Tofu Chickpea Dipping Sauce (page 185), or Sweet
White Sesame Seed Soya Dressing (page 187), to serve

1 Fill a large bowl with cold water and add some ice cubes
   and salt, then set aside. Put the carrots in a steamer over
   boiling water and cook for 5 minutes or until crisp-tender.
   (Alternatively, in a microwave steamer, microwave the carrots
   for 1–2 minutes on full power – or according to the steamer/
   microwave instructions – until crisp-tender.)

2 Plunge the carrots into the iced water, to stop them cooking.
   Remove them and pat dry with kitchen paper. Repeat with
   the cauliflower, peppers, peas and radish. Serve the steamed
   vegetables and the tomatoes with sauces to dip.

Stocks

Dashi, Japanese cooking stock, is the heart and soul of the Japanese cuisine. It adds umami, savoury – the fifth taste (the other
four: sweet, sour, salty and bitter). For many Japanese dishes,
dashi unlocks a unique, subtle, unforgettable layer of flavour,
delicately wrapping around and enhancing the other four tastes
and ingredients' natural flavours.

Dashi can be substituted with Western-style cooking stocks such
as no-salt-added vegetable, meat or fish stock, depending on
what a recipe calls for and what works for you.

Dashi is best made right before use. It can be stored in a refrigerator and freezer, but the aroma and flavour will diminish over
time.

Vegetarian Shiitake Mushroom Dashi Cooking Stock

Use this savoury and earthy vegetarian stock for any dish that calls for cooking stock. Makes 450ml (16fl oz)

> 10 dried shiitake mushrooms, rinsed

1   Put the shiitake mushrooms in a medium saucepan. Add 500ml (18fl oz) water to the pan, bring to the boil and immediately turn off the heat. Leave the mushrooms to rest in the liquid for 15 minutes.

2   Pour the stock through a fine-meshed sieve lined with muslin. Drain the shiitake mushrooms, then squeeze them gently to remove the excess water. Cut off and discard the stems. Use them in another recipe (see Tip). Store the stock in an airtight container in the fridge for up to five days.

> TIP Dehydrated mushroom caps (once pre-soaked) can be used in a variety of dishes, such as soups, sautéed vegetables, simmered vegetables and noodle sauce (page 157).

Fish and Sea Vegetable Dashi, Cooking Stock – First Dashi

This is the most widely used cooking stock for Japanese cuisine. The first dashi is best suited for clear soups because of the clarity of the broth. It also has a more pronounced flavour, which enhances the other ingredients it is cooked with. Makes 1 litre (1¾ pints)

> 1 kombu sheet, 10cm (4in) square
> 25g (1oz) large bonito flakes

1   Do not wash or wipe off the whitish powder on the kombu's surface; it contains natural minerals and adds flavour. Put the

kombu in a medium saucepan. Add 1 litre (1¾ pints) water and bring almost to the boil. Immediately remove the kombu (saving it for making the second dashi, below) to avoid the liquid becoming bitter.

2 Add the bonito flakes and heat the liquid over a high heat until boiling, then immediately turn off the heat and leave the flakes to rest in the liquid for 2 minutes. Pour the stock through a fine-meshed sieve lined with muslin. Avoid pressing on the flakes, to prevent the stock becoming cloudy and bitter. Save the bonito flakes for the second dashi. Leave to cool and store in the fridge for up to two days (it spoils quickly) or freeze for up to three weeks.

Second Dashi Stock

Makes 1 litre (1¾ pints)
used kombu and bonito flakes from First Dashi

1 Combine the used kombu and the bonito flakes from making the first dashi in a medium saucepan. Add 1 litre (1¾ pints) cold water and bring the mixture to the boil. Reduce the heat to low and simmer for 10 minutes. Pour the stock through a fine-meshed sieve lined with muslin, and discard the solids. Leave to cool and store in the fridge for up to two days.

Instant Dashi

As a quick alternative, you can use instant dashi Japanese cooking stock sold at a Japanese grocer's. It comes in the forms of dried seasoning flakes or granules. Please read the packet label to make sure that it contains no salt, monosodium glutamate (MSG) or other artificial ingredients. Each form and brand differs in its preparation and use, so please read the directions on the packet.

Salad dressings, dipping sauces and condiments

Sweet Dashi–Soy Seasoning Sauce

The seasoning sauce is a must-have: a wonderful, instant season-ing in your back pocket. Make ahead and store in a refrigerator for up to one week. Makes 750ml (26fl oz)

    1 kombu sheet, 10cm (4in) square
    500ml (18fl oz) low-salt soy sauce
    250ml (9fl oz) hon-mirin
    2 tbsp sugar
    25g (1oz) large bonito flakes

1   Put the kombu in a medium saucepan, and add the soy sauce. Heat over a medium heat. Add the hon-mirin and sugar. Gently stir to mix the ingredients and dissolve the sugar. Bring almost to the boil, then immediately remove the kombu.

2   Add the bonito flakes and heat the liquid over a high heat until boiling, then immediately turn off the heat and leave the flakes in the liquid for 2 minutes. Pour the sauce through a fine-meshed sieve lined with muslin. Avoid pressing on the flakes, to prevent the sauce becoming cloudy and bitter.

Sesame Oil Salad Dressing

This nutty, aromatic, low-acidity dressing, with a touch of sweetness, is gentle yet flavourful for children. It brightens up everyday salads and gives them a subtle, intriguing dimension. Makes 100ml (3½fl oz)

    3 tbsp rice vinegar
    ½ red onion, finely chopped
    1 tsp brown sugar

1 tbsp toasted sesame oil
sea salt and freshly ground black pepper

1   In a small bowl, whisk together the vinegar, red onion and brown sugar until the sugar has dissolved. Whisk in the sesame oil and season with a generous pinch of salt and several grinds of pepper.

Traditional Japanese Sweet Vinegar Dressing

This is an all-purpose, basic Japanese vinegar dressing. It is elegant and subtle. Perfect for tossing into salads, and drizzling over gently steamed vegetables and grilled or steamed seafood and meat dishes. Makes 250ml (8fl oz)

125ml (4fl oz) brown rice vinegar
2½ tbsp hon-mirin
125ml (4fl oz) dashi (first or second dashi) (page 182)

1   Mix the vinegar and hon-mirin in a small saucepan, and add the dashi. Bring almost to the boil over a medium heat, then remove from the heat and cool to room temperature. Store in the fridge for up to one week.

Creamy Tofu and Chickpea Dipping Sauce

Children love dips for finger foods. Hand them a variety of colour-ful, gently steamed vegetable sticks and let them go wild with this finger-licking yummy dipping sauce! It makes a wonderful snack for birthday parties and playdates. Makes about 225g (8oz)

100g (3½oz) canned chickpeas, drained and rinsed
85g (3oz) soft/silken tofu
1 tbsp lemon juice
4 tsp extra virgin olive oil

1   Put all the ingredients in a food processor or blender and blend until smooth. Serve or store the sauce in an airtight container in the fridge for up to two days. Serve with toasted bread fingers or Lightly Simmered Crudités (page 180).

Toasted and Ground Flaxseeds

Use these as an all-purpose omega-3-rich, nutty and aromatic condiment for any dish. You can also add it to baking flour mixtures. It is easy to toast flaxseeds, but you can also buy them ready toasted if you prefer.

40g (1½oz) flaxseeds

1   Put the flaxseeds in a dry frying pan over a low heat. Swirl, or stir, the pan slightly above the stove to move the seeds around so that they toast evenly. Continue to swirl and/ or stir the seeds for 10 minutes or until golden brown and shiny.

2   Grind the toasted seeds in a seed grinder, or using a mortar and pestle. Store in an airtight container in the fridge and eat within 1 month. You can also store the toasted seeds and grind as much as you need just before you use them, for a fresher taste.

Toasted and Ground White Sesame Seeds

Use this for Sweet White Sesame Seed Soy Sauce Dressing (page 187) and as an all-purpose healthy, aromatic condiment for noodles, sautéed vegetables, salads and tofu dishes. It is easy to toast and grind sesame seeds at home, and the results are better, but you can also buy them ready toasted and ground for convenience.

40g (1½oz) white sesame seeds

1   Put the sesame seeds in a dry frying pan over a low heat. Swirl, or stir, the pan slightly above the stove to move the seeds around so that they toast evenly. Continue to swirl and/or stir the seeds for 10 minutes or until golden brown and shiny.

2   Grind the toasted sesame seeds in a grinder, or using a mortar and pestle. Store in an airtight container in the fridge and eat within 1 month. You can also store toasted seeds and grind as much as you need right before you use them, for a fresher taste.

Sweet White Sesame Seed Soy Sauce Dressing

This dressing is traditionally used to flavour gently boiled or steamed spinach. The sweet, tangy and nutty sauce delights children and makes vegetables more delicious. See a sample recipe for Tender Vegetables with Sweet Sesame Seed Dressing on page 177. Makes 200ml (7fl oz)

40g (1½oz) Toasted and Ground White Sesame Seeds (see above)
1½ tsp low-salt soy sauce
1½ tsp sugar
a pinch of salt

1   Put all the ingredients in a small bowl and stir together well.

Sweet Red Miso Sauce

This is a savoury and sweet dip that goes well with practically anything: vegetables, tofu, seafood and meats. See a sample recipe for Aubergines and Red Peppers with Sweet Red Miso Sauce (page 174). Makes about 2 tbsp

2 tbsp dashi
2 tbsp reduced-salt red miso
2 tsp sugar

1   Put all the ingredients in a small bowl and stir together well.

All-purpose Vegetable Tomato Sauce

Make a batch of Japanese Sweet Potato, Pumpkin, Bean and Tomato Soup (page 141), blend a portion of it and pour it into ice-cube trays. Cover with clingfilm and freeze. Use the cubes of sauce for pizzas (page 143) and pasta sauces for young children. It is more substantial and nutritious than shop-bought tomato-based sauces. Make ahead so that you have it for last-minute meal preparations. Makes 300ml (10fl oz)

> 300ml (10fl oz) Japanese Sweet Potato, Pumpkin, Bean and Tomato Soup (page 141)

1   Put the soup into a blender or food processor and blend until smooth. Pour the mixture into ice-cube trays. Cover with clingfilm and freeze for up to one month.

Leafy Green Vegetable Ice Cubes

Use these vegetable cubes to increase the vegetables in snacks and meals, especially for children who are reluctant vegetable eaters. See sample recipes on pages 189 and 190. Makes 500ml (17fl oz)

> 300g (10oz) frozen chopped spinach and/or kale
> a few drops of lemon juice
> 150g (5½oz) frozen carrots
> 1 tbsp ground flaxseeds

1   Put the ingredients and 125ml (4fl oz) cold water into a blender or food processor and blend until smooth. Pour the mixture into ice-cube trays. Cover with clingfilm and freeze for up to one month.

Bakes and snacks

Chia Seed and Chocolate Chip Cookies

Adding chia seeds to a dish is a wonderful and super-convenient way to boost your intake of the heart-healthy omega-3s and other nutrients such as fibre – plus, it has a delicious texture. For these cookies, I like to use kinako – roasted soya flour – which is often used in traditional Japanese confectionary. It has an earthy, toasted aroma and flavour, as well as containing protein. Other secret ingredients are fruits and leafy greens for natural sweetness and nutrients. This recipe is egg-free because sometimes I need to make egg-free snacks for our son to take to school or camp when a classmate is allergic to eggs. Or sometimes, once I've started cooking I realise that I don't have any eggs (oops!). I find improvising makes cooking all the more fun! Makes about 48 mini-cookies

40g (1½oz) plain flour
35g (1¼oz) wholemeal flour
37g (1⅓oz) kinako roasted soya bean flour
¼ tsp bicarbonate of soda
1½ tsp chia seeds
100ml (3½fl oz) olive oil
50g (1¾oz) dark brown sugar
50g (1¾oz) caster sugar
½ tsp salt
1 tsp vanilla extract
½ ripe banana, mashed
1 tbsp grated apple, or ready-made apple sauce
1 ice cube Leafy Green Vegetable (see page 188), thawed
½ tsp kudzu (Japanese arrowroot), or arrowroot or potato starch, dissolved in ½ tsp water
70g (2½oz) milk chocolate chips

1   Preheat the oven to 190°C/375°F/Gas 5. Line 2 baking sheets with baking parchment or a non-stick silicon baking mat. Sift the flours and bicarbonate of soda into a bowl and add the chia seeds. Combine well.

2   Put the oil, sugars, salt and vanilla in a large bowl and, using a handheld or stand mixer, or a large rubber spatula, mix at a medium-low speed for 30 seconds or until fully incorporated. Add the banana, apple and vegetables, and mix for 1 minute or until the mixture is smooth.

3   Gradually stir in the flour mixture, stopping once or twice to scrape down the side of the bowl using a flexible spatula, until well combined. Slowly add the kudzu water while beating at a slow speed. Stir in the chocolate chips, and stir until all the ingredients are well incorporated.

4   Scoop out half of the dough, roll into balls and put 24 on a baking sheet. Bake in the centre of the oven for 10–12 minutes, rotating the sheet halfway through, until the cookies are golden brown. Cool on the sheet for 8 minutes and then transfer the cookies to a wire rack to cool to room temperature. Repeat with the remaining mixture.

Brown Rice and Kinako Soya Flour Mini Muffins

My family loves these mini-muffins. I batch-bake and freeze them. They are perfect for a quick breakfast, on-the-go snacks, and an instant hunger satisfier between meals. They have been big hits among our family friends with small children. And best of all, my son eats vegetables this way. Makes 24 mini-muffins

240g (8½oz) unsalted butter or 240ml (8½fl oz) rapeseed or olive oil, plus extra for greasing
a pinch of sea salt
3 large eggs
3 Leafy Green Vegetable Ice Cubes (page 188), thawed
2 tsp vanilla extract

200g (7oz) caster sugar or 185ml (6fl oz) amber agave
65g (2¼oz) brown rice flour
30g (1oz) kinako roasted soya bean flour
130g (4¾oz) wholemeal flour

1   Preheat the oven to 160°C/325°F/Gas 3 and lightly grease 24 muffin cups.

2   Put the butter or oil in a large bowl and sprinkle with the salt, then set aside. Put the eggs in a small bowl and mix in the thawed vegetables and vanilla extract. Set aside.

3   If using butter, beat it using a handheld or stand mixer, or a large rubber spatula, until creamy. Slowly add the sugar to the butter or oil, while beating the butter or stirring the oil, until smooth and fluffy.

4   Add the egg mixture slowly, while beating or stirring, occasionally scraping down the inside of the bowl. Sift the flours over the mixture in three batches and fold each in using a rubber spatula until combined.

5   Pour the batter into the prepared muffin cups, and bake for 20–30 minutes until golden brown and crispy on the edges. Test using a cocktail stick or a skewer. If it comes out clean, the cakes are done. If not, bake for another 5–10 minutes. Cool the muffins in the pan on a wire rack for 15 minutes, then remove from the pan and leave them to cool completely on the rack. Serve warm with tea or milk.

Fruit and Vegetable Smoothie

A home-made fruit and vegetable smoothie is truly so much more delicious and nutritious than shop-bought milkshakes, slushes or ice creams, because it is loaded with fruit and two secret ingredients – leafy greens and flaxseeds – and no-added sugar or artificial flavours. The sweet fruit helps the leafy greens go down. Smoothies make delightful snacks for children after outdoor play, sports or a swim. They also make an instant waker-upper breakfast for teenagers and grown-ups on busy mornings, especially on hot days, when appetites might be a bit low. Frozen fruit makes it a snap to create a thick, slushy texture. I use shop-bought frozen peaches, berries and mangoes, because they are economical and convenient, but you can also slice and freeze fresh fruit in season if you are unable to buy a variety of frozen fruit. I also alternate between different types of milk to vary the flavours. I like soya milk for its subtle sweetness and silky tone. If serving dairy milk to children under five, use whole milk (see Appendix III). Makes 450ml (16fl oz)

1 ripe banana, peeled
a few drops of lemon juice
250g (9oz) frozen peaches or fresh peaches, sliced and frozen
a small handful of frozen chopped spinach or kale
⅓ small frozen or fresh carrot
125ml (4fl oz) whole milk or soya milk
1 tbsp ground flaxseeds

1   Put the banana into a blender or food processor then blend until smooth. Add the lemon juice and the remaining ingredients, and blend again. Serve immediately in a wide-mouthed glass, cup or a bowl with a spoon.

Speedy bites and teas

The simplest foods make great snacks for children. Try:

• Edamame beans – simmer 75g (2¾oz) frozen shelled edamame beans in boiling water for 5 minutes or until crisp-tender. Drain in a colander. (Alternatively, microwave the frozen edamame in a microwave-safe bowl for 1–2 minutes – or according to the microwave instructions – until crisp-tender.)

➡

- Drained and rinsed canned chickpeas, and raw mangetouts.

- Sliced bananas on thin toasted multigrain/wholegrain bread, or white bread for under-fives.

- Slices of cheese, such as mild Cheddar or firm mozzarella, with thinly sliced apple. Dip the apple slices in lemon juice water, drain and pat dry so that they won't discolour.

- Fresh seasonal fruits are hassle-free and taste great – strawberries, raspberries, cherries, peaches, nectarines and plums – as well as grapes, bananas, melons, mangoes and many more that are available almost all year.

Caffeine-free unsweetened barley teas

Cold mugicha Put 1 mugicha tea bag in 1 litre (1¾ pints) cold water and leave to infuse for 2 hours in the fridge or according to the directions on the packet.

Hot mugicha Put 1 mugicha tea bag in 1.5 litres (2¾ pints) boiling water and leave to infuse for 3–5 minutes or according to the directions on the packet.

5

Healthy-eating Inspirations

The Japanese diet shares similarities with a number of traditional diets from around the world. All of them celebrate the food patterns that have been eaten for many generations. The modern diet today in the UK has moved away from traditional ways of eating and this may be a chief contributor to chronic disease. We can learn a great deal from societies who have retained their traditional ways of eating.

The food-and-nutrition education organisation, Oldways, aims to guide people towards good health through heritage. Their website (see www.oldwayspt.org) includes several helpful food pyramids for healthy eating, which show the proportions of different types of foods as they would be traditionally eaten in certain areas of the world, such as the Mediterranean and the countries of Asia.

Their Asian Diet Pyramid was developed in conjunction with the Cornell-China-Oxford Project on Nutrition, Health and Environment, and the Harvard School of Public Health. The traditional diet in many Asian countries is often closely tied to religious practices and long-standing customs, and the record of eating habits is an excellent source of information and culinary inspiration.

The Asian diet's geographical base includes countries like Japan, China, Indonesia, Malaysia, South Korea, Singapore, Taiwan, Thailand and Vietnam. Although each country and region has its distinct flavours and cooking styles, almost all share one food in common: rice, which is prepared and eaten slightly differently from country to country. As the staple food central to survival, especially during times of famine, rice has acquired an almost sacred status in Asian societies. It is served in many ways and is a significant part of many meals. Although many Asian food cultures are based on white rice, health authorities urge us to choose more nutrient-rich whole-grain options like brown rice.

Another unifying characteristic of the traditional Asian diet is a high consumption of plant foods – including vegetables, fruits and legumes (peas, beans and lentils). When Asians give up these traditional foods for a more Western diet, however, their health can plummet. Diabetes rates in China, for example, today rival those in the United States, and obesity and overweight are soaring as fast food and sedentary lifestyles replace a life of manual labour fed by rice and vegetables.

Whether you choose familiar vegetables, fruits, grains and other foods and flavour them with Asian spices, or experiment with less-familiar ingredients from an Asian market, you'll find plenty of delicious choices if you are interested in incorporating a more Asian angle into your diet.

Whatever food patterns your family enjoys, remember that a varied diet, which includes all the food groups, is essential, and that it is especially important to give children a good balance of healthy foods to help them grow physically and mentally.

Appendix I

Expert opinion: the early years

By Leann L. Birch and William P. 'Bill' Flatt, Professor, Department of Foods and Nutrition, The University of Georgia and Leading Authority on Healthy Children's Eating.

These suggestions [the 'seven secrets to nurture a healthy child' in this book] are all excellent, and give guidance about what to do rather than what not to do – phrasing them positively is the way to go.

However, the very early period of life, when the bulk of the transition to the adult diet occurs, has been largely ignored in the (scientific) literature. I would argue that by that time many dietary patterns are well established.

That doesn't mean that they can't be changed, but it's easier to establish new patterns than to change old ones.

I do think there are also a few don'ts to go with the do's – such as the importance of limiting children's access to sugar-sweetened beverages, including juice, and not using food to control children's behaviour, including using food to soothe and deal with non-hunger distress. The 'do' here is to learn to recognise and distinguish hunger from other distress, while using other soothing strategies for non-hunger distress, and learning to recognise and respond appropriately to the child's fullness cues. For example, parents of infants can use swaddling, white noise, rocking, non-nutritive sucking (pacifier [dummy]) with an infant who is fussy but not showing signs of being hungry. Our own work suggests that parents of infants and toddlers who use food to soothe and fail to distinguish hunger from other distress or don't recognise fullness cues tend to overfeed, which can result in excessive weight gain, a risk factor for later obesity. This provides yet another rationale for breastfeeding, because it is difficult to overfeed a breastfed infant, as the infant plays an active role in the feeding process. In contrast, it is very easy to overfeed an infant who is being bottle fed – whether it's formula or breast milk or something else such as juice in the bottle.

Finally, learning to enjoy a variety of healthy foods also starts early – Julie Mennella's [biopsychologist at the Monell Chemical Senses Center in Philadelphia] work and our own shows that infants readily learn to accept and like the foods and flavours that are offered to them, thereby learning to like and eat the foods in the local diet. If the mother is breastfeeding, the infant becomes familiar with many flavours of the local diet, because they appear in her breast milk.

The devil is in the details as usual; encouraging children to eat foods that compose a healthy diet is challenging because young children tend to be 'neophobic' and reject new foods and flavours when they are first offered, unless they are sweet or salty – preferences for those tastes, as well as umami, appear to be unlearned.

Parents need to understand that initial rejection doesn't mean that the child will never accept the food – they should persist with repeated, 'no pressure' opportunities for children to try a small taste of new foods.

With this approach, many of those new foods will be accepted and liked, but sensitive, responsive parenting is needed to pull this off.

Appendix II

Expert opinion: be your child's role model

By Prof. Anoop Misra, Chairman, Fortis-C-DOC Centre of Excellence for Diabetes, Metabolic Diseases and Endocrinology, Chairman, National Diabetes, Obesity and Cholesterol Foundation (N-DOC), Director, Diabetes and Metabolic Diseases, Diabetes Foundation (India) (DFI) and Dr Seema Gulati, Head, Nutrition Research Group, Centre of Nutrition & Metabolic Research (C-NET), National Diabetes, Obesity and Cholesterol Foundation (N-DOC), Chief Project Officer, Diabetes Foundation (India).

Being very strict is only going to increase the craving for junk food. Flexible restraint works better because it teaches children self-discipline, which helps them throughout their lives.

It is important for all the family members to engage themselves in some physical activity such as going for walks together, playing some sports, swimming, dancing or any other physical activity. It not only strengthens family ties but it also motivates children and parents to continue their physical activity.

As we have seen, family oriented meals are associated with healthier eating habits in children. Mothers often determine the feeding environment and food-related attitudes, and they influence the child's ability to self-regulate their intake.

Parents should be role models for their children. If parents are enjoying fried food and sweetened beverages, it will be wrong to expect their children to consume healthy foods.

Family environment and eating habits are very important in determining the food choices of children. In our recent study on dietary habits of mothers and children, we observed a high degree of overlap between the dietary intake of mothers and their children. [Gulati, S., Misra, A., Colles, S.L., Kondal, D., Gupta, N., Goel, K., et al. 'Dietary intakes and familial correlates of overweight/obesity: A four-cities study in India', *Annals of Nutrition and Metabolism*, July, 2013.]

Patterns of food choice of mothers and their children showed an extremely high level of overlap in our recent study. Marked similarities between food and nutrient intake within families have also been reported. Parents have a vital role to play, especially as the food procurer and preparer, in shaping the types and amounts of food children consume. Research studies suggest that poor parental modelling, a less authoritative parenting style, and fewer family-oriented meals are related to increasing child BMI.

It is important for all the family members to maintain a healthy weight through improving food choices, increasing physical activity and reducing television and recreational computer time.

Appendix III

Feeding guidelines for infants and young children

This book focuses on children aged 5 to 12. The World Health Organization recommends the following guidelines for infants and young children: 'Early initiation of breastfeeding within one hour of birth; exclusive breastfeeding for the first 6 months of life; and the introduction of nutritionally-adequate and safe complementary (solid) foods at 6 months together with continued breastfeeding up to two years of age or beyond. Complementary foods should be rich in nutrients and given in adequate amounts. At six months, caregivers should introduce foods in small amounts and gradually increase the quantity as the child gets older. Young children should receive a variety of foods including meat, poultry, fish or eggs as often as possible. Foods for the baby can be specially prepared or modified from family meals. Complementary foods high in fats, sugar and salt should be avoided.' (World Health Organization, October 2014.)

How much salt do babies and children need?

Babies and children need only a very small amount of salt in their diet; however, because salt is added to a lot of the food you buy, such as bread, baked beans and even biscuits, it is easy to have too much.

The maximum recommended amount of salt for babies and children is:

up to 12 months – less than 1g of salt a day (less than 0.4g
   sodium)
1 to 3 years – 2g of salt a day (0.8g sodium)
4 to 6 years – 3g of salt a day (1.2g sodium)
7 to 10 years – 5g of salt a day (2g sodium)
11 years and over – 6g of salt a day (2.4g sodium)

Babies who are breastfed get the right amount of salt through
breast milk. Infant formula contains a similar amount of salt to
breast milk.

When you start introducing solid foods, remember not to
add salt to the foods you give to your baby because their kidneys
cannot cope with it. You should also avoid giving your baby
ready-made foods that are not made specifically for babies, such
as breakfast cereals, because they can also be high in salt.

Lots of foods produced for children can be quite high in salt,
so it's important to check the nutritional information before you
buy. The salt content is usually given as figures for sodium. As a
rough guide, food containing more than 0.6g of sodium per 100g
is considered to be high in salt. You can work out the amount
of salt in foods by multiplying the amount of sodium by 2.5. For
example, 1g of sodium per 100g (3½oz) is the same as 2.5g salt per
100g (3½oz).

You can reduce the amount of salt your child has by avoiding
salty snacks, such as crisps and biscuits, swapping them for low-
salt snacks instead. Try healthy options such as dried fruit, raw
vegetable sticks and chopped fruit to keep things varied.

Fibre

As explained in Secret 1, the NHS advise that children under five
do not have wholegrains such as pasta, wholemeal bread and
brown rice, as it is too filling and leaves no room for the more
nourishing foods. Wholegrains can be gradually introduced
after this age. Fibre in the form of vegetables and fruit is,
however, recommended for children under five years. For more

information see: http://www.nhs.uk/conditions/pregnancy-and-baby/pages/baby-food-questions.aspx#close

Weight and BMI

To check if your child's weight falls into the healthy range, see: http://www.nhs.uk/Tools/Pages/Healthyweightcalculator.aspx

Index